Springer Series on MEDICAL EDUCATION

SERIES EDITOR: Steven Jonas, M.D.
SERIES ADVISERS: Howard S. Barrows, M.D. • John Gordon Freymann, M.D. • David Rabin, M.D., M.P.H.

VOLUME 1 Problem-Based Learning: An Approach to Medical Education
Howard S. Barrows, M.D., and Robyn M. Tamblyn, B.Sc.N.

VOLUME 2 The Evaluation of Teaching in Medical Schools
Robert M. Rippey, Ph.D.

VOLUME 3 The Art of Teaching Primary Care
Archie S. Golden, M.D., M.P.H., Dennis G. Carlson, M.D., M.P.H., M.A., and Jan L. Hagen, M.S.W., *Editors*

VOLUME 4 Medical Education in the Ambulatory Setting: An Evaluation
Loyd J. Wollstadt, M.D., Sc.M., Dennis A. Frate, Ph.D. and Mark G. Meyer, M.A.T.

VOLUME 5 Teaching Preventive Medicine in Primary Care
William H. Barker, M.D.

VOLUME 6 The Interpersonal Dimension in Medical Education
Agnes G. Rezler, Ph.D., and Joseph A. Flaherty, M.D.

VOLUME 7 Assessing Clinical Competence
Victor R. Neufeld, M.D., FRCP(C), and Geoffrey R. Norman, Ph.D., *Editors*

VOLUME 8 How to Design a Problem-Based Curriculum for the Preclinical Years
Howard S. Barrows, M.D., FRCP(C)

VOLUME 9 Implementing Problem-Based Medical Education: Lessons from Successful Innovations
Arthur Kaufman, M.D., *Editor*

VOLUME 10 Clinical Teaching for Medical Residents: Roles, Techniques, and Programs
Janine C. Edwards, Ph.D., and Robert L. Marier, M.D., FACP, *Editors*

Janine C. Edwards, Ph.D., received her doctoral degree in instructional design from Florida State University in 1979. She has a background in teaching, administration, and development of curricula and training programs in school systems and industries. Presently she is Coordinator, Office of Educational Development and Evaluation, and Research Associate Professor of Medicine, at the Louisiana State University School of Medicine in New Orleans. Her research interests include graduate medical education, faculty development, and evaluation in clinical settings.

Robert Marier, M.D., FACP, received his medical degree from Yale University School of Medicine, New Haven, CT. He completed a residency in internal medicine at Massachusetts General Hospital, Boston, and a fellowship in inflammatory diseases at Yale University. He was appointed Assistant Professor of Medicine at Yale before relocating to the Louisiana State University School of Medicine in New Orleans, where he is now Professor of Medicine. He has served as Program Director of the Residency Training Program in Internal Medicine at LSU and Associate Medical Director at Charity Hospital in New Orleans.

Clinical Teaching for Medical Residents

Roles, Techniques, and Programs

Janine C. Edwards, Ph.D.
Robert L. Marier, M.D., F.A.C.P.
Editors

Springer Publishing Company
New York

Springer Publishing Company, Inc.
536 Broadway
New York, NY 10012

88 89 90 91 92 / 5 4 3 2 1

Library of Congress Cataloging-in-Publication Data

Clinical teaching for medical residents.

(Springer series on medical education ; v. 10)
Bibliography: p.
Includes index.
1. Medicine, Clinical—Teacher training. 2. Residents (Medicine)—Training of. I. Edwards, Janine C. II. Marier, Robert L. III. Series.
R833.5.C57 1988 610′.7′11 87-28554
ISBN 0-8261-5600-2

Printed in the United States of America

We dedicate this book to the residents of the Louisiana State University School of Medicine in New Orleans, who have taught us so much about the process of clinical teaching.

Contents

Preface

The goal of this book is to provide support and develop the role of teaching for residents within the established priorities of residency training. The resident's medical training comes first, patient care is second and instrumental to the development of clinical competence, and teaching is third. A few general observations about residents and the general health care (medical education) environment are in order, because we must work within this context.

The role of the house officer in the life of the medical school and hospital has been visualized classically as one of learner and provider of services. Resident physicians, along with medical students, were seen as receivers of the teaching efforts of attending staff and of faculty conference leaders. Their own role as teachers, until recent times, was not formally recognized. Now the importance of the resident as teacher is being increasingly appreciated. Medical schools have recognized the large number of valuable contact hours between residents and students, and the fertility of the teaching environments in which daily interaction occurs between these co-learners.

Medical centers in the past have done relatively little to prepare residents for teaching medical students. How we may best teach residents to teach in the traditional as well as the developing ambulatory environment poses a major challenge to medical educators. Principles for resident teaching in all clinical settings are evolving.

Residents differ in their affinity and ability to teach (Tonesk, personal communication). A few residents teach well intuitively; they usually also have higher than average clinical competence. Most residents, although willing to teach, need assistance to develop good teaching skills. This majority will benefit from training in teaching skills. Some residents have little or no interest in teaching; they require motivation to fulfill their responsibility and to acquire training in teaching skills. Finally, a few will not develop good teaching techniques despite efforts to train and motivate them.

Residents work under a great deal of stress, and they have responsibility for teaching. Without support and guidance to fulfill the teaching role, stress increases. Residents require support for other aspects of their lives as well. Personal and family support services are needed, as are financial and career-planning support. Slowly these needs are being recognized.

Today's broad economic and political changes are forcing increased attention on graduate medical education. Containing costs of health care is a major problem. The federal government has forced this issue by establishing Diagnostic Related Groups (DRGs). Although the full effect of DRGs on medical education is not yet known, the trend is clearly toward decreasing money for medical education. Faculty of medical centers are feeling economic pressure to generate more revenue to support themselves and their institutions (Perry et al., 1981). These societal changes lead to a decrease in the amount of time that faculty members have to teach. The traditional role of teaching students, then, can be expected to take on added importance for residents.

Finally, we emphasize the broader nature of teaching skills for residents' benefit. Because physicians must teach patients to prevent disease and comply with treatment, the teaching skills residents learn can be useful throughout their lives. The broad interpersonal skills that are learned in teaching students transfer to interactions with patients.

The objectives of the book are to: (1) provide practical advice and resources about clinical teaching and its evaluation, and about teaching improvement programs for residents; (2) stimulate recognition of the resident's teaching role; and (3) give perspectives from research and theory for future development of teaching techniques, evaluation, and improvement programs.

The book is organized in three parts. Part I presents information about the roles of residents as learners and teachers and the developmental stages of a resident's professional growth.

Steward and Feltovich (Chapter 1) present the goal of learning as development of professional competence, which has three attributes: a knowledge base, problem-solving strategies, and a disposition toward self-improvement. The authors also explain why the residents' intermediate position in the medical education hierarchy is helpful. Residents may be more understanding of students' concerns and may communicate more easily with them than do faculty. Residents' thought processes are more similar to students' thought processes than are those of faculty members. Residents benefit from teaching by acquiring skills they can use not only with students during training, but also with patients and other health care professionals throughout their careers.

Stritter and his associates (Chapter 2) explain a major theory within which residents' teaching should be viewed: developmental psychology. The most important difference between attending physicians and residents is that the latter are developing their skills and knowledge base. They are physicians in training. Throughout their training, they are growing intellectually and emotionally. Developmental psychology holds important practical implications for resident teaching, which Stritter has outlined. Integrating teaching principles, which are abstract concepts, into concrete experience with students is important. Spacing instruction about teaching throughout the months when teaching responsibilities are heaviest is another practical consideration that is stimulated by recognition of residents' developmental characteristics.

Part II gives practical techniques for teaching in clinical settings, lecturing, and evaluating teaching. Also in Part II, methods for improving teaching are reviewed, theoretical perspectives for future development are presented, and research methods for studying clinical teaching are explained.

A chapter on Sir William Osler presents the case for exemplifying that great physician as a clinical teacher par excellence. Knight (Chapter 3) presents those personal and professional characteristics that make Osler an enduring figure; his ideas about relating to students and patients, bedside teaching, learner independence, and setting priorities; and his passions—for books and medical history. Osler's thoughts and life are inspirational, and Knight's anecdotal style approximates the warm, enthusiastic, energetic personality of his subject.

Edwards and Marier (Chapter 4) present practical teaching techniques for inpatient and outpatient settings. Their sources of information include research; experts' opinions; perceptions of students, attending physicians, and residents; and adaptations of social science theory and research. The following techniques are described: plan ahead, win cooperation, communicate objectives, use patients, think aloud, build a knowledge base, set a good example, motivate, give feedback, and evaluate. Emphasis is given to teaching the complex skills of problem-solving and clinical procedures.

Whitman (Chapter 5) sets forth the types of learning that can be achieved in lectures: learning of facts and understanding interrelationships and applicability of those facts. This chapter describes techniques for attracting and maintaining attention during a lecture: questioning, brainstorming, demonstrating, role-playing, and problem-solving. Whitman also offers advice about the delivery of lectures, including audiovisual aids, speaking voice, and body movements. This information can serve residents well throughout their lives, because the lecture is a standard method of teaching in the medical profession. Whitman's lively style stimulates interest in his subject.

Skeff and his associates (Chapter 6) review methods for improving teaching and present guidelines based on educational and psychological theories for teaching improvement programs. Methods for improving teaching include student and peer evaluation, consultation with an educator, videotape review, self-evaluation, concept-based training, and multicomponent methods (seminars and workshops). The multicomponent methods have been shown to be more effective than the single-component methods. The relative effectiveness of each element within multicomponent methods is not known, however. Furthermore, the fit of resident teaching improvement methods to various institutional settings has not been tested empirically. To supplement existing knowledge, the authors present 18 questions drawn from theories to guide persons in developing resident teaching improvement programs.

Irby (Chapter 7) gives some pragmatic advice about incorporating evaluation of teaching into the total residency program. He points out that the teaching role, as well as the clinical competence, of residents should be evaluated because this reinforces the value of teaching. Irby describes the purposes of evaluation, seven criteria for teaching excellence, and four strategies for evaluating. Guidelines for developing rating forms and tips on managing an evaluation system are given.

Weinholtz (Chapter 8) thoughtfully reviews studies of attending physician teaching and proposes a series of three studies of residents' clinical teaching. The first two studies are designed to answer the question, "What is effective clinical teaching by residents?" The last study would determine whether participation in a teaching improvement program enhances resident teaching. In the first study, Weinholtz proposes that a large number of ward teams be observed, each for 2 weeks, by a research team. He explicates steps in conducting such observations.

The second study would correlate teaching behaviors with learner outcomes. Resident work rounds would be observed to collect information about low-inference teaching behaviors, contexts, and locations. Weinholtz proposes correlating student ratings of resident teaching with the observed data.

In the third study, an educational consultant would give feedback from observation to individual residents about their teaching. This would be an experimental study with treatment and control residents.

Part III includes case studies on the development of teaching improvement programs for residents. These case studies illustrate concretely the successes and problems that medical centers have encountered in trying to improve resident teaching. They yield valuable lessons for other institutions interested in developing such programs. The final chapter highlights themes drawn from throughout the book.

This book will have fulfilled its goal when teaching is widely recognized as an integral component of the resident's clinical competence, and training and evaluation of teaching skills are routinely included in residency programs.

Acknowledgments

We acknowledge with gratitude the seminal role that Paul F. Larson, M.D., has played in initiating the teaching improvement program at Louisiana State University and, ultimately, in the development of this book. He had the foresight in the early 1980s to begin a program for training residents in teaching skills, and he gave the full weight of his authority as Dean of the Louisiana State University School of Medicine in New Orleans to making the program successful. Dr. Larson was instrumental in institutionalizing the residents' teaching skills program. Our studies of resident teaching and this book are products of his support. We appreciate his personal encouragement and guidance throughout our work.

Special thanks are due to Dr. Xenia Tonesk, former staff member of the Association of American Medical Colleges, who suggested that we produce a book to foster the teaching role of residents. She gave impetus to the project and encouraged us throughout its review. Her diplomatic guidance at critical points assisted in bringing this work to fruition. We also acknowledge the encouragement of other staff members of the Association of American Medical Colleges who reviewed and supported the initial proposal.

The National Fund for Medical Education has provided support for a number of programs described in the case studies and for clinical teaching studies conducted by contributing authors of other chapters in this book. Their broad contribution to the development of clinical teaching is gratefully acknowledged.

We are grateful to Charles F. Chapman, Coordinator of the LSU Medical School Editorial Office, for his expert assistance and advice throughout the process of preparing the manuscript. His guidance contributed significantly. Juliette Scott and Angela Stewart gave invaluable help by typing, proofreading, and preparing computer files of the manuscript. Finally, we thank Dr. Julie Brannan, our research assistant, who contributed in numerous ways to development and evaluation of our program as well as to proofreading the manuscript.

Contributors

Judith Berman, Ph.D., received her doctorate of education from the University of Massachusetts, Boston, with emphasis on research in educational psychology. Her past work has included family studies and human relations training. Presently she is Co-Director of the Stanford University Faculty Development Program, Palo Alto, CA.

Steven Borkan, M.D., is a Research Fellow in Nephrology at Boston University Medical Center. He completed his residency training in internal medicine at Michael Reese Hospital and Medical Center, Chicago, where he also served as Chief Resident. He was formerly Director of the General Medicine Consultation Service at Michael Reese Hospital.

Martha G. Camp, Ph.D., is the Associate Director, Offfice of Educational Research and Services, at the Bowman Gray School of Medicine of Wake Forest University, Winston-Salem, NC. Holding a doctorate in science education, she has drawn on her background as a teacher and her study of the learning process in the initiation of several innovative programs for faculty and students at the Bowman Gray School of Medicine.

Paul J. Feltovich, Ph.D., is an Assistant Professor, Department of Medical Education, at Southern Illinois University School of Medicine. He received his doctorate in educational psychology from the University of Minnesota in 1981 with an emphasis on problem-solving and cognitive skill development in complex fields, including medicine. His current work is studying the role of basic biomedical science knowledge in the clinical reasoning and performance of physicians.

Rhonda M. Goldberg, M.A., is the Director, Office of Education, of the George Washington University School of Medicine and Health Sciences in Washington, DC. In addition to her responsibilities in the areas of curriculum, evaluation, and student affairs, she regularly conducts workshops for faculty, residents, and students to help them develop their skills as teachers.

Larrie W. Greenberg, M.D., is Professor of Child Health and Development, George Washington University School of Medicine and Health Sciences, and has been Director of Medical Education at the Children's Hospital National Medical Center in Washington, DC, since 1978. Besides his clinical and administrative duties, his research interests have focused on teaching, learning, and career counseling.

J. Dennis Hoban, Ed.D., has been the Director, Office of Educational Research and Services, at Wake Forest University's Bowman Gray School of Medicine, Winston-Salem, NC, since 1978. His major interest is the teaching/learning process in formal and informal teaching settings. In addition to his educational interests, he has been increasingly involved in cost-containment intervention research.

David M. Irby, Ph.D., is Associate Professor in the Division of Research in Medical Education and Assistant Dean for Planning at the University of Washington School of Medicine in Seattle. Over the past 15 years he has worked on the evaluation and improvement of teaching in medical education. Dr. Irby has conducted over 200 faculty development workshops nationally and internationally, conducted research on clinical teaching in medicine, developed teaching evaluation systems for medical schools, published a book and several articles on the evaluation and dismissal of medical students, and served as a consultant to medical schools here and abroad. He earned a doctorate in education from the University of Washington in 1977 and completed a postdoctoral fellowship at Harvard Medical School in 1983.

Leslie S. Jewett, Ed.D., is Assistant Professor of Allied Health and Development at the George Washington University School of Medicine and Health Sciences, and Associate Director, Office of Medical Education, at the Children's Hospital National Medical Center, Washington, DC. She is also Director of the Division of Continuing Medical Education within the Office. Her research interests have been in teaching, learning, and career counseling.

James A. Knight, M.D., is Professor of Psychiatry and Medical Ethics at the Lousiana State University School of Medicine in New Orleans. He is active in the American Osler Society and the Society for Health and Human Values, organizations involved in the history of medicine and the humanities in medicine. Throughout his professional life, Dr. Knight has been deeply involved in resident and medical student teaching, both at the bedside and in the classroom and laboratory.

Linda Lesky, M.D., is an Assistant Professor of Medicine at Boston University School of Medicine. Currently the Associate Director of the General Medicine Group Practice and Chief of the Women's Health Group at Boston University Medical Center, she was formerly the Medical Director of the Portes Center of Chicago and Director of the Internal Medicine Clinic at Michael Reese Hospital and Medical Center in Chicago. She was also formerly a member of the Educational Development Unit at Michael Reese Hospital, where she completed a Medical Education Fellowship.

William D. Mattern, M.D., is a Professor of Medicine and Associate Dean for Academic Affairs of the School of Medicine at the University of North Carolina at Chapel Hill. His scholarly interests are nephrology, renal dialysis, clinical education, and clinical instruction.

Franklin Medio, Ph.D., is an Associate Professor of Medical Education in the Division of Educational Resources at The Chicago College of Osteopathic Medicine. In this position, he serves as the evaluation specialist and the coordinator of faculty development for the College. His research interests include clinical teaching and evaluation, patient–physician communication, and the use of "simulated patients" for faculty development. He was formerly a member of the Educational Development Unit at Michael Reese Hospital and Medical Center in Chicago.

C. Benjamin Meleca, Ph.D., is Professor and Director, Division of Research and Evaluation in Medical Education, at The Ohio State University College of Medicine. In addition to educational training programs for faculty and house staff, he is interested in academic affairs, curriculum development, and evaluation.

James A. Pearsol, M.Ed., has a background and training in educational psychology. He is a research associate in the Division of Research and Evaluation in Medical Education at Ohio State University, Columbus. His primary interests are in educational program planning and evaluation.

Edward J. Shahady, M.D., is a Professor of Family Medicine at the University of North Carolina at Chapel Hill. He was formerly Chairman of the Department of Family Medicine at UNC and President of the Society of Teachers of Family Medicine. His academic interests include clinical education, clinical teaching, sports medicine, and the application of the principles of family medicine.

Kelley M. Skeff, M.D., Ph.D., is a member of the Division of General Medicine at Stanford University and Assistant Chief of the Department of Medicine at the Palo Alto Veterans Administration Medical Center. He received his Ph.D. in education from Stanford University in

1981. His research has focused on the development and evaluation of teaching improvement methods for attending physicians. He is Director of the Primary Care Faculty Development Program at Stanford.

David E. Steward, M.D., is a general internist on the faculty of the Southern Illinois University School of Medicine, Springfield. He is the Director of the Ambulatory Medicine Program, Chairman of the Clinical Competence Committee for the Internal Medicine Residency Program, and Director of the Introduction to Clinical Medicine course for second-year students.

Georgette Stratos, Ph.D., received her Ph.D. in educational psychology from the University of California at Berkeley in 1981. She is a Research Associate in the Division of General Medicine at Stanford University, conducting research in medical education. Currently she is Co-Director of the Stanford University Faculty Development Program, Palo Alto, CA.

Frank T. Stritter, Ph.D., is a Professor in the Schools of Medicine and Education at the University of North Carolina at Chapel Hill. He is also Director of the Office of Research and Development in Education for the Health Professions. His professional interests include curriculum, instruction, clinical education, and faculty development.

Donn Weinholtz, Ph.D., is an Associate Professor in the College of Education and an Assistant Research Scientist in the Office of Consultation and Research in Medical Education at the University of Iowa. His research interests are describing effective teaching by attending physicians, especially during attending rounds, and developing and evaluating methods for improving attending physician teaching.

Neal Whitman, Ed.D., is an Associate Professor and Director of Educational Development in the Department of Family and Preventive Medicine at the University of Utah School of Medicine, Salt Lake City. He has been an administrator, teacher, and consultant in medical education since 1971. His academic interest is in the improvement and evaluation of teaching, and he is particularly interested in the role of the resident as a teacher.

LuAnn Wilkerson, Ed.D., is the Director of Faculty Development at Harvard Medical School, Boston. As Director, she is responsible for working with faculty in the New Pathway Program. Her research interests include the application of problem-based learning to clinical teaching, selection and training of tutors, and the impact of curriculum change on faculty. She was formerly a member of the Educational Development Unit at Michael Reese Hospital and Medical Center, Chicago.

PART I

Resident Roles

CHAPTER 1

Why Residents Should Teach: The Parallel Processes Teaching and Learning

DAVID E. STEWARD
PAUL J. FELTOVICH

Residents are teachers. For the reader, this statement may seem obvious and unnecessary. You know that residents teach, and that in general they do so competently and effectively. They teach at the bedside during work rounds; they give short or long lectures in the hallway as needed and as time permits; they teach critical thinking in the middle of the night when there is no one else to do so; they spend hours reading and critiquing write-ups for students; they conduct textbook-review seminars to ensure that students learn a systematic approach to clinical practice; they present topics at department or subspecialty conferences or rounds; they organize board-review courses to teach themselves; and they teach by example when they become unwitting but appropriate role models for innocent medical students. In many in-

Preparation of this chapter was supported in part by a grant from the Josiah Macy Jr. Foundation.

NOTE: Throughout this book, the pronouns "he," "his," and "him" should be understood to refer to persons of either gender, unless specific gender is clearly indicated.

stitutions, residents do the bulk of the basic clinical teaching of students and junior residents, especially in the inpatient setting.

It is no accident that clerkship and residency directors encourage and even demand so much teaching from residents. First, for teaching medical students, no one is more available or better qualified than a resident. Furthermore, teaching is simply a good thing for residents to do. On one level, as part of their basic training residents should acquire and practice teaching skills that they may find useful during their later professional lives. On another more important level, residents learn a lot as they teach. They expand their knowledge base, they learn to use their knowledge creatively in helping students solve clinical problems, and one can even say that when residents teach they learn how to learn.

As programs are developed to help residents do more and better teaching, those planning the programs must understand the place of residents in the educational process. In this chapter, we first examine the nature of the learning process as it pertains to the students that residents teach and to residents themselves. Then we examine the goal of learning—the professional competence that residents are trying to achieve in their education. We next consider residents as teachers with specific attention as to why they are in a good position to help students learn. Finally, we examine the benefits from teaching that residents accrue toward their *own* learning, emphasizing the relationships between teaching, learning, and the development of professional competence.

RESIDENTS AND STUDENTS AS LEARNERS

That students are in medical school to learn is self-evident. Although it is important for them to teach, residents also participate in residency training programs primarily to learn. Learning, an active process by which one modifies one's own knowledge, abilities, or behavior, typically occurs in response to some current situation. For example, another person, such as a teacher, may pose a question that one cannot answer, or a circumstance in daily professional activity may arise for which one is not prepared. For residents and students, the situation is likely to be a patient with a problem that must be evaluated and managed. The importance of the situation motivates the person to find a solution, and the process of learning is begun.

The Learning Process

Although the specifics for each situation and individual may vary, the learning process comprises three general steps, especially when learning involves complex and difficult subject matter, as is typical in medicine (Champagne et al., 1985; Glaser, 1984; White, 1983).

1. The learner must focus attention on what he already knows or can do regarding the problem. This focusing may not be as easy as it would seem. A learner may not want to face the inadequacy of his existing knowledge or ability, and therefore may avoid thinking about it. In addition, complicated concepts or those used infrequently may be difficult to retrieve. Furthermore, some knowledge may actually be tacit—one may have knowledge but not be fully aware of it. Despite the difficulties, one must clearly understand preexisting knowledge and abilities before deficiencies can be identified and modifications made.
2. Once knowledge or skills pertinent to an issue are identified, inappropriate aspects must be challenged. The learner or teacher formulates such a challenge by comparing what is needed for resolution of the current situation to what is already known or to skills that can already be carried out. The result, in educational terms, is the identification of learning issues or objectives (Barrows, 1983). These objectives may be specific (e.g., which enzyme digests dietary proteins in the small bowel?) or general (e.g., how should heart failure be managed?); they must be clear enough to direct learning.
3. Finally, the learner must engage resources that can provide information or advice needed to resolve the learning issues and solve the problems. For a resident, available resources might include an expert physician who is making rounds, books or journal articles, lectures or seminars, or even colleagues. For the student, a useful resource is often the resident. A resource must have available the facts needed by the learner and must be accessible, reliable, and concise. In addition, the learner must know how to use the resource properly.

These three steps are useful to everyone when they learn. Not everyone is good at them, however, nor does everyone do them routinely or comfortably. These steps require skill to be successfully executed and, as with any other skill, practice and guidance may be needed to develop and master them. Poor performance of any of the steps will lead to ineffective learning of complex material. For residents and students to be effective learners, then, they must practice and perfect these steps as a routine part of their training. But what are residents and students trying to learn?

The Goal of Learning: The Development of Professional Competence

The details of what residents and students should learn vary considerably and depend on many factors such as the particular specialty, the faculty, the patient population, and the resident's or student's personal goals and wishes. To avoid the complications that might be produced by trying to specify exactly what residents should learn, we will use "the development of professional competence" as the general goal of all kinds of medical training, and discuss how this process occurs.

The term "professional competence" defies a simple definition. It refers to a complex and multifaceted talent or ability that enables a physician to efficiently and reliably approach and solve the wide variety of clinical problems that may arise in the practice of medicine. Professional competence involves more than learning a trade, more than perfecting technical skills, and more than applying algorithms to common presenting situations. Physicians must be prepared to deal with vague problems, arbitrary time constraints, incomplete and possibly unreliable information, and ill-defined goals that may change as a problem progresses. The professional competence that enables physicians to manage in the face of these inconsistencies has three important cognitive attributes: an extensive, flexible knowledge base; efficient expert problem-solving strategies; and a disposition toward ongoing improvement of both knowledge and problem-solving.

Knowledge Base

There is no substitute for knowing a lot. Specialist physicians must know enough to understand clinical problems at multiple levels, from molecular and cellular levels through the levels of the whole patient and even society in general. They must be able to manipulate their knowledge and use it creatively to solve clinical problems that are never exactly the same. Residents and students acquire such a rich and flexible knowledge base by repeatedly encountering and using pertinent information in a variety of ways. When residents and students actively use and manipulate information, rather than passively encounter it, they will learn it more effectively. Residents and students are relatively passive when they are exposed to information in seminars, lectures, and general textbook and journal reading. Residents and students use information actively when they encounter it in the course of patient care.

Expert Problem-Solving Strategy

Reflecting novice and expert problem-solvers more generally (Chi et al., 1981), novice *clinical* problem-solvers approach clinical problems differently from experts (Feltovich et al., 1984). Novices (e.g., medical students) break a problem down into component parts and analyze each part separately. They then attempt to combine the results of all of the analyses to arrive at some final solution. In contrast, experts (e.g., faculty members) assemble the components of a problem to form a pattern of information and associated interpretations. As a result of their experience, experts can recognize such data patterns as indicators of specific diagnoses, diagnostic clusters, and solutions without having to analyze each part of the problem separately. Expert problem-solving strategy is more efficient than the novice strategy, and because it requires fewer analytical steps, the expert approach is less prone to operational errors. With the ultimate goal of achieving expertise, residents are "developing experts"—their approach is intermediate between students and faculty members.

Ongoing Improvement of Knowledge Base and Problem-Solving Strategy

A professionally competent physician keeps up with advances in medical science and technology by routinely using the three learning steps described above, through which the knowledge base and problem-solving strategy can be readily modified. The professionally competent physician must apply this cycle of steps as a regular part of daily life, and not as an occasional special event. Residents and students acquire the ongoing self-improvement habit if they develop the skills of self-assessment, are willing to acknowledge when they do not know something, are helped to identify the most effective resources available, and are held responsible for learning as a result.

For any person, the three cognitive attributes of professional competence discussed above develop gradually over time and to different degrees. What comprises normal or abnormal development is a complex question to which there are no clear answers. Trainees, however, may have identifiable deficits in one or more of these attributes that may improve with specific educational interventions. For example, a resident with a weak knowledge base may benefit from directed reading assignments with specific rigorous evaluations of what he learns as a result. Or, a resident perceived to be inflexible may have problems improving ongoing problem-solving strategies; he might improve through careful, repeated challenge of the problem-solving process by an appropriate expert. The way that professional competence develops may also influence how residents should teach. For example, individual residents with significant deficits in any of the attributes should have limited teaching responsibilities, and the general level of development of groups of residents at different stages of training should influence the overall design of clinical teaching programs.

Having discussed the general process of learning and the goals of learning for both residents and students, we can turn to the special place of the resident in the teaching process.

RESIDENTS AS TEACHERS

In their clinical years, medical students frequently consider their most important teachers to be the residents with whom they regularly work. Students may be more in awe of the attending physician who makes rounds three times a week; they may think they hear more "pearls" from the fellow; they may find the subspecialty consultant to be a great source of detailed information; and they may find seminars, lectures, and grand rounds to be useful in learning about selected topics. But they usually recognize that they learn the real basics of clinical medicine through the teaching and guidance of residents.

How Residents Teach

When residents teach, they attempt to help students with the learning steps described earlier in the chapter. In some circumstances, such as lectures or case conferences, there is little interaction and students simply listen passively to what the resident has to say. In most teaching done by residents, however, such as during hospital rounds, clinical conferences, or day-to-day patient-care activities, the resident and student interact a great deal, and teaching and learning occur in a dynamic tutorial fashion. This style of teaching is particularly powerful in engaging (and conveying to students) the three-step cycle of learning (Collins and Stevens, 1982).

The common scenario for this kind of teaching is as follows: The resident and one or more students are involved in the evaluation and management of a patient. The overriding goal is to provide patient care, but the resident also must use the situation to teach students. There are many variables in each specific situation, such as the levels of development of the resident and the students, the difficulty of the problem, and whether the problem is managed in a single episode (e.g., the outpatient setting) or in several episodes (e.g., the inpatient setting). Despite this complexity and variation, the resident guides the students through the three steps of the learning process. First, the resident must determine what the students already know. Students may simply volunteer what they know; it may be apparent from how they write orders, present a case, or perform a procedure; or the resident may need to question them directly. Next, the resident must help students challenge their knowledge and develop learning issues. Students should have somewhat different learning issues than the resident in most cases—which learning issues are whose must be clearly understood. Finally, the resident must help students identify and use pertinent resources. The resident may suggest several alternatives, such as textbooks, lectures, or expert faculty members, or the resident may take it on himself to be a resource. The latter can be a profitable option for both students and the resident—the student's learning needs are directly addressed in a timely and focused fashion, and the resident must review and rethink pertinent parts of his knowledge or problem-solving strategy to explain them to students.

Thus, through resident teaching, students learn not only the knowledge and problem-solving strategies needed to evaluate clinical problems; under the guidance and modeling of the resident, they also begin to acquire the learning skills they will need for their own professional competence.

Why the Resident Can Be a Particularly Good Teacher

Why are residents so likely to be effective and influential teachers? We propose two general reasons. The first one is simple—residents are the most available persons capable of doing clinical teaching. They are around all of the time, even through the night, and they participate in all aspects of the care of patients, including emergency care, triage and admitting, routine inpatient evaluation and management, and discharge planning. Without residents, either clinical faculty would need to be available to teach on a 24-hour-a-day basis, a radical new source of clinical teaching would be necessary, or the clinical teaching to which students have become accustomed would not get done. None of these three alternatives seems likely, and, therefore, residents are needed to teach simply because they are in the right places at the right times.

The other reason residents are good teachers is this: Their knowledge, authority, and experience are more than those of the student or junior resident but less than those of the faculty member. This intermediate position is desirable on several counts. One is that students are less intimidated by residents than by most faculty members and are willing to open up to residents, ask questions, and demand teaching when it is needed.

A second benefit of the resident's intermediate position is that, because residents have themselves been students relatively recently, they understand better than faculty members the practical needs and problems of students. Thus, residents take seriously students' concerns about the call schedule, upcoming exams, writing orders, or starting IVs, whereas faculty members may consider such concerns inconsequential or silly.

A third benefit is that students are likely to be able to communicate better with residents than with faculty members about clinical problem-solving. As we have discussed, novices (e.g., students) and experts (e.g., faculty members) approach problems differently. Novices analyze the individual component parts of a problem separately, while experts assemble component parts into a broad pattern of information and interpretations. As a result, when they attempt to discuss clinical problems, students and faculty members may have conflicting perspectives and priorities—students are likely to want guidance in understanding details of problems and their implications, while faculty members are attuned to more global, integrated considerations. The difference may be exacerbated by tendencies toward tacitness that occur with highly practiced skills such as those of the expert (Schneider and Shiffrin, 1977); the expert may lose conscious access to some of the underlying bases for what he does. As developing experts, residents occupy a useful niche between the two approaches. Although they have more clinical expertise than students, residents are still likely to understand students' approaches to and concerns about clinical problems and be better able to communicate with them about these things. At the same time, residents can carefully and incrementally lead the students toward the more expert approach. If students try to hasten the process and adopt expert methods (such as large associative leaps over causal mechanisms) before they have mastered the basics, they may end up with faulty clinical reasoning processes that do not serve as a healthy foundation for the development of true clinical expertise (Lesgold et al., in press). By understanding students and guiding them through the process of development, residents can play a critical role in helping students lay the groundwork for future professional competence.

HOW THE RESIDENT BENEFITS FROM TEACHING

Although the intended beneficiaries of resident teaching are the students who are being taught, the residents who do the teaching are themselves benefited in several ways. Obviously, they acquire teaching skills that they will use for the rest of their careers. Less obviously, but perhaps more importantly, as residents teach, they improve their own knowledge bases and problem-solving strategies, and they develop learning habits and skills needed to maintain lifelong professional competence.

Acquisition of Teaching Skills

Teaching skills can be valuable for the practicing physician in many professional activities, perhaps the most important of which is patient education. The three basic steps of teaching that are acquired and used by the resident to teach students can be used by the practicing physician to educate patients effectively. As applied to patient education, the first step of the process—finding out what the patient knows or believes about his medical condition—is critical. Patients often have health beliefs that are not based in biomedical principles, but rather are nonscientific or mystical in origin. The physician must obtain clear understanding of what a patient believes to decide what information to provide to the patient and how to provide it. In addition, the use of all three steps in a dynamic, tutorial-style interaction between physician and patient, similar to that between resident and student, improves the physician–patient relationship and promotes patient compliance (Eraker et al., 1984). Although residents must develop patient education techniques while dealing with patients, the skills they acquire while teaching students are consistent with and directly applicable to the patient education process.

Physicians may have many other uses for good teaching skills. For example, they may be called on to speak to lay groups, service organizations, or schoolchildren; they may be asked to present seminars or to be teachers for hospital conferences or continuing medical education programs; and they may serve as clinical faculty for medical students, residents, and fellows. These activities are important services that physicians routinely provide to the community and the profession, and they are also opportunities for physicians to promote themselves to colleagues and the public.

Teaching, Learning, and Professional Competence

Development of Knowledge Base

Teaching helps residents develop the broad, rich, flexible knowledge base that the competent physician must have to approach and solve unique clinical problems. The resident–teacher constantly reviews, reorganizes, and uses what he knows as each of the three steps of the teaching process is executed. During the first step, as the students are helped to display what they know, the resident must use his own knowledge as a reference to judge the accuracy and adequacy of students' knowledge. The resident must build a flexible knowledge base to make these judgments appropriately, because individual students may have cognitive structures for storing, organizing, and retrieving knowledge that differ from the structures used by any other student or by the resident. During the second step, as the resident–teacher helps students challenge their existing knowledge, the resident must again use his own knowledge in a creative way to pose challenges that are clearly understood by students and that help students develop appropriate learning objectives. And, in the third teaching step, when the resident serves as a resource for students, he must organize and present his knowledge so that students can comprehend and use it to satisfy their own learning objectives. Thus, the activities required during each of the teaching steps help the resident–teacher develop a flexible, usable knowledge base that can be creatively applied to any situation, including clinical problem-solving.

In addition to promoting flexibility and creativity, teaching helps the resident expand and broaden the knowledge base. Challenges or questions from students may lead a resident to discover deficiencies in what he knows. Such challenges can be deflected and rendered useless if the resident tells the student to "look this up for yourself." However, if residents are encouraged to be good teachers, a student-generated challenge can be a strong stimulus to a resident to learn new information, both to correct his own deficiency and to satisfy students. Furthermore, students may trade roles with the resident and serve as resources themselves. They may possess particular knowledge as a result of previous education or experience, or they may respond to learning objectives developed *with* the resident by researching pertinent issues and reporting findings during later discussions. There are pitfalls in the student resource—a resident may rely too much on students as resources and not develop his own learning skills, and students may become disenchanted if they think they are being taken advantage of. In general, however, the student resource can be helpful to the busy resident who may not have time to read or get to the library.

Development of Expert Problem-Solving Strategies

Just as it helps a resident develop his knowledge base, teaching can enhance the resident's development of reliable and consistent expert problem-solving strategies. In the same way that the knowledge base is

CHAPTER 2

The Resident as Professional and Teacher: A Developmental Perspective

FRANK T. STRITTER
EDWARD J. SHAHADY
WILLIAM D. MATTERN

Here presented is a model that can guide a program for development of medical residents as professionals and as teachers. The model describes the professional development of a resident so that clinical instruction can be designed to influence it. *Professional development* is the process of change in which learners are engaged as they gradually assume the characteristics of a practitioner in their chosen field. Those characteristics are developed during an educational program pursued under the auspices of a department within a school of medicine or an external site such as a community hospital affiliated with a school. *Clinical instruction,* which facilitates that development, is the interaction between instructor/practitioner and learner that normally occurs in the proximity of a patient and focuses on either the patient or a clinical problem associated with the patient (Stritter and Flair, 1980). The number of learners dealt with at any one time is small, generally not exceeding three or four, and the "patient" can be viewed as an individual, a family, or a community. Clinical instruction has important consequences because of the responsibilities eventually assumed by those being taught for the health care of a given population.

Underlying the model is the assumption that a resident develops professionally in a series of sequential stages, each necessitating more complex behavior than the previous one. Each stage results from a growth in learning the complex information, skills, and sensitivities comprising a physician's role. In certain respects, these stages are similar to, but not identical to, the developmental stages in a child's thinking as described by Piaget (1963). Current theories of development assume universal achievement of stages, spontaneous acquisition of characteristics, and an invariant sequence and hierarchical integration of stages in the process, all of which occur without special environmental intervention (Feldman, 1980). Learning, as evidenced by medical residents in a formal educational program, includes that additional portion of human development that results expressly from environmental intervention supplemented by individual study and reading, from teaching and counseling by more advanced residents and attending physicians, and by the practical experience of both taking care of patients and teaching those in a clinical setting who are less mature. What a resident does both formally and informally, therefore, must be included in the formula explaining his development as a physician and as a teacher.

Viewing a resident's development from a stage perspective has significant educational implications. It can provide an analysis of a resident's educational encounters with his clinical instructors and conclusions about their success or failure as stimulants for learning. It can also help to assess the configuration of a resident's abilities at each stage and suggest what can be done to improve or otherwise facilitate his development.

A DEVELOPMENTAL PERSPECTIVE

In his development as a professional physician, a resident progresses through a series of successive structural stages. Each resident has certain characteristics that change in discernible ways as he passes through those stages and becomes more mature in his professional role. A developmental model assumes that a resident's behavior both as a learning physician and as a teacher of himself, of medical students, and of less mature residents is governed by an internal mediating process that evolves structurally according to the resident's collective experiences at a given time.

Several dimensions or multiple traits of professional development are apparent. One could say that an approach similar to a factor analysis, but with intuitive values instead of hard data to support its conclusions, assisted us in specifying those dimensions of professional development. The dimensions were then organized by us into a map of traits explaining a resident's progress from one stage to another. Each trait has its own developmental trajectory and course, but all traits seem to become interdependent as the resident matures.

According to Sprinthall and Thies-Sprinthall (1983), the assumptions of a developmental theory are that: (1) humans process their experience through cognitive structures called stages, (2) such stages are organized hierarchically from the less complex to the more complex, (3) growth occurs first within a particular stage and then only to the next stage in the sequence, (4) growth is not automatic but occurs only with appropriate interaction between the learner and his environment, and (5) a learner's behavior can be explained by determining his particular stage of development.

Early credit for thinking about learners from a cognitive–developmental perspective can be attributed to Dewey:

> The aim of education is growth or development.... Ethical and psychological principles can aid ... in the greatest of all constructions—the building of a free and powerful character. Only knowledge of the order and connection of the stages in psychological development can insure this. Education is the work of supplying the conditions which will enable the psychological functions to mature in the freest and fullest manner. (Dewey, 1970)

In designing a model that documents the educational and professional development of medical residents, one must recognize that physicians continue to learn throughout their productive years, that learning does not cease on completion of a basic educational program. Furthermore, one must recognize that as a learner matures in his professional role, he (1) evolves his learning focus from abstract concepts to the concrete problems that he faces in the clinical setting, (2) applies what he learns immediately as opposed to at some future time, (3) increasingly uses his personal experiences as the basis for his own learning, and (4) increasingly orients his learning to the tasks he perceives to comprise his future professional role. This personal orientation leads to a conclusion that each resident passes through specified stages during his own time frame and that both instruction and assigned responsibilities based on the resident's particular stage facilitate his clinical learning.

THEORIES OF HUMAN DEVELOPMENT

The view of adult development as a progression through a series of stages is not new, but its application to the growth of medical residents may be. Theories most relevant to the medical residency portion of adult development describe that growth in various ways. "Cognitive growth" during childhood and adolescence was charted by Piaget (1963). His model of intelligence emphasizes the development of biologically based structures that produce qualitative changes in the way one functions cognitively as the individual matures. In relating his theory of stage development to adults, Piaget (1972) pointed out that each adult has the capacity for attaining a certain stage in his intellectual capabilities on the condition that the social environment and experience provide him with intellectual nourishment and stimulation. Such achievement also depends on the person's aptitude and professional specialization. One's stage of development at any given time is, therefore, contingent on both individual characteristics and environmental conditions.

"Ego development" is an approach to viewing human development as conceptualized by Loevinger (1976). The various stages in one's ego development constitute qualitatively different frames of reference for perceiving and responding to oneself and one's relationship to other people. It is that aspect of one's personality that strives for personal coherence by assigning meaning to one's experience and determining one's responses to it. Loevinger suggests that an individual reaches various levels depending on education and degree of sophistication. As one develops, the sense of self is first governed by fear of retaliation and external pressure, next to a conformity to outside rules, later to living by self-evaluated standards, then to self-determination of those standards and respect for one's own individuality, and finally to an integrated stage that adds reconciliation of inner conflicts in a consolidated sense of personal identity. One's particular stage at any given time provides the framework of the perspective for viewing relationships and experiences, including education, and assigning them value and meaning.

Another version of development is offered by Kohlberg (1976) in his description of "moral development." Individuals are constantly faced with ethical dilemmas in which they must decide on courses of action by virtue of their moral judgment. Kohlberg sees that one's ability to make those decisions changes as one passes through six stages. Within each successive stage in this personal conception of justice a hierarchical reorganization of the moral concepts of the preceding stage occurs, leading to a more complex understanding of an ethical dilemma and then to a more just resolution for that person. Moral development is traced through various stages in the understanding of the concept of human rights and through a systematic expansion in the universe of people who are considerations in making a moral judgment. At each successive stage, the universe to which moral judgments are applied is expanded, leading to a more just decision for all. Kohlberg suggests that not all persons achieve the highest stage, but that those who operate at the higher levels of moral development tend to function at a more competent level in other areas of their lives.

Yet another form of development, "ways of knowing" or learning, was researched and later described by Perry (1970). Although Perry's research focused on college students and their patterns of thought, his rationale can be applied to many other levels of learners. Learners reinterpret their lives and their views of the world in each successive stage. Learners move from familiar patterns of meanings and acquiring knowledge that are comfortable or that perhaps fail them to new patterns, where they begin to make sense of broadening experiences that nonetheless threaten them with new implications for their lives. As the patterns evolve, learners move to new stages that both include and transcend earlier ones. Perry further defined this evolving way of knowing as acquiring new cognitive strategies available to learn a particular task or skill, or to acquire knowledge from one's environment.

Viewing growth and change in those becoming professionals as development is not, therefore, a new concept. Knowledge from the social sciences contributes to an understanding of the factors that influence development of desirable professional characteristics. This knowledge can be adapted to the development of medical residents, and then perhaps it will become more feasible to develop educational programs and assign responsibilities that maximize that development.

THE PROFESSIONAL DEVELOPMENT OF A MEDICAL RESIDENT

In Figure 2.1, the horizontal axis of the "Learning Vector" refers to the professional development of the individual resident. When he first enters the clinical setting, the resident can be considered a novice relative to that particular experience. As his contact with and exposure to the setting increases, the learner becomes more and more mature. He progresses from principles to application, from absolutes to relatives, and from single to multidimensional responses to the stimuli in his environment. That maturational development can be classified in three stages of professional development. First is *Exposure,* beginning in

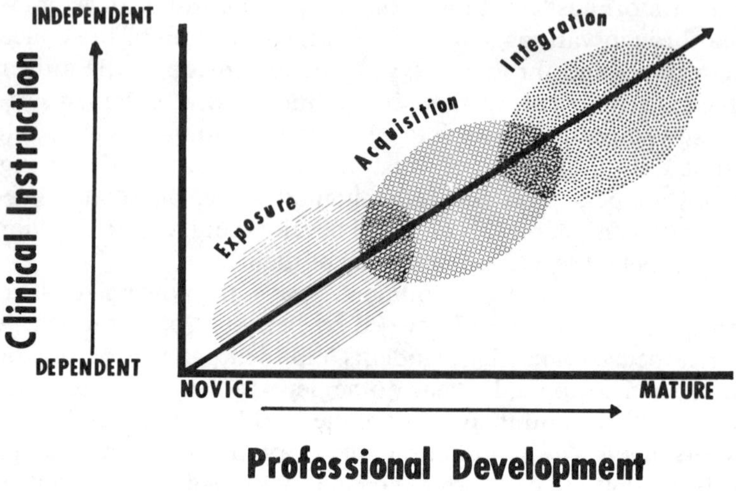

FIGURE 2.1 Professional development: The learning vector.

medical school and continuing into residency, as a learner is merely exposed to basic facts, information, concepts, and attitudes from a variety of sources presented to him in new ways (e.g., an attending physician, preceptor, a patient, a host of other health professionals, and even the environment). Residents may not be aware that they are learning things that will shape their future roles as physicians and clinical teachers. Second is *Acquisition,* in which the resident tests the given information, concepts, skills, techniques, and styles by applying them in his clinical responsibilities. He now begins to focus on making decisions and reasoning. Third is *Integration,* in which the learner weaves the acquired characteristics into a personal professional identity that he perceives can launch him on his medical career. It involves his final pursuit and attainment of a comfortable professional style.

Specific dimensions comprise that personal development or maturation at each stage. The resident exhibits each of the dimensions, but in different ways that depend on his particular state of development. First is the *cognitive*—the information or knowledge base coupled with both intuitive and analytical reasoning that allows the professional to use that base (Piaget, 1972). Second is the *technical*—the physical and manipulative skills that enable the professional to ascertain information about his patients and/or to conduct various procedures (Posner and Keele, 1973). Third is the *attitudinal*—the interests, values, and ethics that guide resolution of moral problems, action, choice of behavior, argument, and rationalization (Rokeach, 1979; Sheehan et al., 1980). Fourth is *psychosocial*—those characteristics of interpersonal and human interaction that underlie sensitivity to and communication with patients and fellow health care team members (Havinghurst, 1972). Fifth is *socialization*—the internalization of professional values and the commitment of professional role (Bucher and Snelling, 1977). Sixth is *independent learning*—that allows a professional to stay current with the changing sciences of his field (Knowles, 1970). The final characteristic is his ability to *teach* other learners in the environment (e.g., medical students, less advanced house officers, other health professional students).

During the first, and possibly the second, stage of development, each of the seven dimensions progresses and evolves relatively independently from the others, with the developmental lines being jagged and uneven. The technical skills and the information base develop first. Cognitive skills such as reasoning develop later and add to enriched technical ability. Psychosocial skills develop more as the resident gains in understanding his patients' physical and emotional problems. Professional and life experience help the resident build his psychosocial skills and contribute to the development of attitudes. At the end of the second and during the third stage, the dimensions begin to merge and finally become inseparable. Development and/or modification of any single dimension now influences development and/or modification of all the others. They have become interdependent. Thus, the fully mature physician is better able to help his patients because he understands their problems from all dimensions.

THE EXPOSURE STAGE: A RESIDENT'S EARLY PERSONAL CHARACTERISTICS AND TEACHING RESPONSIBILITIES

In the exposure stage, a resident observes his peers, attending physicians, or preceptors, becoming more aware of basic information, skills, and attitudes that are demonstrated in the clinical setting and that will be necessary to possess in an eventual professional role.

Regarding the cognitive dimension, the young doctor views many practices of patient care implemented by more advanced residents and supervising faculty members. His observations of more experienced physicians stimulate recall of knowledge from his medical school courses. For example, a knee examination can help the resident remember the anatomy of bones, cartilage, muscles, and ligaments that comprise the knee. He is completely immersed in care of individual patients by actually having to provide immediate care to a panel of patients. He practices care based both on what he remembers from more casual medical student encounters with similar patients and on what he sees his peers doing. He is asked to comment on any aspect about a particular patient and feels he must be a fountainhead of information about that patient. The resident's own questions concern the immediate differential diagnosis and management needs of that patient, although there is no time for reading about the nature of that patient's problem and its relation to the principles of pathophysiology. He, therefore, does what he can to find out critical information about his assigned patient(s) and to have it available for specific questions asked by his superiors.

Pertaining to techniques, the resident is exposed to technicians and others who deliver life support and critical care to his patients using skills such as cardiopulmonary resuscitation. He will be asked questions about the implementation of what he sees and may even be expected to perform the more simple procedures such as chest compression, lumbar puncture, or starting an IV under the watchful eye of the technician or his supervisors.

Attitudinally, the resident observes attitudes toward specific patients or classes of patients that are evidenced by more advanced residents. For example, a more advanced resident may be repulsed by obese, chronically ill, or odorous patients, and this impacts on the way the young resident begins to identify certain values and interests, only some of which may be desirable. He notices that terminal patients are often avoided on rounds, that laboratory values are emphasized as opposed to social history in making a diagnosis, and that approaches to treatment are stressed much more than is prevention in caring for a patient. The resident then experiences similar feelings of involvement, attachment, or repulsion for his assigned patients. He, therefore, acquires attitudes from observing others and from his own experiences with those for whom he cares.

The resident is a member of a work group, such as a ward team or a clinic staff, with an assigned task. The resident observes the necessity for cooperative and effective functioning of that group, which is enhanced by interpersonal skills and sensitive psychosocial interactions. The respect and sensitivity that characterize the way his superiors relate to each other becomes evident. The resident observes how the group members relate to one another as well as to other health professionals. The resident sees how sensitive questions, such as those identifying sexual preference and suicidal tendencies, are asked, and he begins to notice the impact of the team's effort at communication on the patient's well-being. Particularly, he observes how a health professional's communication skills influence patient compliance.

The process of socialization begins for the resident as he observes the attending physician and senior residents. The resident attends staff meetings and ward rounds, noting how hospital and clinical policies are formulated and carried out. The respect that each participant holds for the other becomes apparent. The resident begins to realize that he is a physician and that a significant degree of responsibility is included in his role.

The resident's learning is driven almost completely by the patients for whom he has responsibility and by the expectations of his superiors for the care of those patients. His observations about a patient's condition, any changes that might occur over time, and questions raised by peers and preceptors stimulate the resident to find applications for selected aspects of the information retained from his years as a medical student. He begins to wonder why most of it is not immediately useful to him, however. Some new information is obtained from attending conferences, rounds, and special lectures, but the acquisition of new knowledge is not a primary activity for this resident. The basic skill being learned is how to employ information to which he has already been exposed, how to make knowledge useful for future encounters with similar types of patients in similar settings. The resident is often unsure of how to proceed with a given problem and will seek as much help from more advanced residents and peers as he can obtain. He depends on them to help him learn.

The resident in the exposure state generally has two types of teaching responsibilities and/or opportunities. First, he is often assigned a third-year medical student who provides assistance to the resident in the care of the specific patients assigned to that resident. The relationship between student and resident is one-to-one and always in the context of a small number of patients' conditions and concrete needs. The resident best teaches technical skills to the student, but the resident is usually so overwhelmed by his own fears of inadequacy that the needs of the student are often overlooked. The model of "see one, do one, teach one" operates at the exposure stage. He gains teaching skills most often by imitation of those who are more advanced and by practice. The second type of teaching is to fellow residents at the exposure stage who need the survival skills necessary to complete this initial stage. This teaching is informal, usually implemented in group discussions or by role model. Often a resident is not even aware that he is teaching his peers how to cope attitudinally, but the outcomes of such peer teaching are often more important than any impact he has on medical students.

THE ACQUISITION STAGE OF LEARNING TO CARE FOR PATIENTS AND TO TEACH

In the acquisition stage, a resident tests the information he has obtained, either from his efforts to apply previously learned concepts concerning patient care or from new experiences that occurred in the exposure stage. As the resident endeavors to ascertain whether physiological and therapeutic principles hold true, he will reinforce some and make mistakes implementing others, both of which provide valuable learning. The resident now begins to schedule more time for reading about those principles and for individual learning of new information as he becomes more efficient in his patient care. He begins to raise questions about optional patient evaluation and management as opposed to providing merely adequate care in an overwhelming clinical context. He begins the process of generalizing his concrete experiences to other patient and health care encounters.

Technically, the resident now practices techniques and procedures having to do with critical care and life support. He is often observed by more experienced members of the team and does make errors. As he learns from his mistakes and the feedback received from those around him, he begins to perfect his technique and to perform the procedures with more confidence.

Attitudinally, the resident continues to develop values, interests, and ethics that will eventually characterize him professionally. He now has an opportunity to see how his personal attitudes toward a specific patient affect that patient. For example, he may come to understand that his sense of repulsion in the presence of a morbidly obese patient is sensed by the patient, causing embarrassment and withdrawal from the patient. He may also feel impotent because a diagnosis cannot be made or because a treatment is not working as planned. A resident's feeling of worth is often related to his sense that the patient's health is improving. Similarly, he is able to experience how his own particular values influence his concern for others on the team. For example, a resident may cooperate with others by volunteering to assist less experienced residents when he has time available. He may also exhibit fairness by volunteering to teach the nurses on the team about the latest treatment for a common medical problem they have encountered. He begins to be objective about the impact that his interests, attitudes, and values have on others.

From a psychosocial perspective, the resident is an active member of the health care team and begins to be involved not only in group membership, but also in leadership of the team. He becomes aware that it is not only critical to participate openly and effectively, but also that it is important to organize, direct, and manage a team. He is not yet permitted to function as the head of the team, but he knows that leadership will soon become his responsibility. He continues to experience situations where he must depend on his interactive capabilities with others, such as nurses, technicians, and consulting physicians. The resident either profits or loses from that capability, making him more aware of the necessity to interact effectively with these individuals. The resident should begin to understand how important it is for a patient to comprehend directions and explanations, but often residents make comments or give instructions to patients that are misunderstood. He often does not comprehend his patient's real reasons for asking a question. For example, a mother's question about her child's fever may be based on a myth about fevers that an experienced physician will discover before answering the question. The developing resident should, however, become aware of responsibility to communicate effectively, and should then experiment with a personal style that facilitates a patient's comprehension and compliance.

The process of socialization continues as the resident realizes the power of his contributions to the organization's smooth functioning. He feels more of a sense of mastery of the skills and knowledge necessary for his role as he achieves a greater degree of autonomy and responsibility. He perceives that he is acting independently and that he does have the responsibility for his actions. Commitment and identity with the profession stem from this sense of mastery that comes from many sources—treatment as an expert by others on the team, a correct diagnosis, seeing a patient improve, or an original contribution of some type. The resident is doing more of what he sees the accomplished physician in his environment doing and, therefore, is gradually becoming more socialized to the role he perceives to be required.

With regard to learning skills, the resident feels more pressure to identify an area in which he can become expert. For some this means being able to ask or answer questions more specifically and more expertly. For others it means thinking about subspecialty training, even though they had not intended to become subspecialized when they entered the program. A resident in this stage tends to spend much time reading and attending conferences to supplement his expertise on the various topics that he thinks could be developed as a special knowledge base. A resident now seeks help with increasing selectivity, exercising control over whom he consults with a problem or question, and exercising judgment in considering any advice he receives. The resident is also developing increasing skill in assessing his own performance as well as the performance of his peers and his preceptors. He compares himself to others and then chooses activities to improve knowledge and skill.

As for teaching responsibilities, the resident in the acquisition stage assumes responsibility for the medical students and first-year residents on the team. Group leadership skills are crucial. He spends his time on the ward or in the clinic with groups of learners. He can direct the team of students and residents by virtue of his responsibility for patients assigned to the unit. The resident organizes work rounds and other direct-contact tasks with the patient. As he obtains more knowledge about who, when, and how to consult for advice with patient management, he teaches that information to those on the team either by the model he demonstrates or by his instructions. He likes to see the junior members of the team supplement their patient experiences with reading, just as he is now doing, but can be frustrated when they focus on spending time with the patient and do not seem interested in reading. The resident in this stage generally has more direct responsibility for teaching than do residents at the other stages.

THE INTEGRATION STAGE: THE MATURE RESIDENT'S PERSONAL CHARACTERISTICS AND TEACHING ACTIVITIES

The resident in the integration stage polishes those characteristics he has chosen for his own professional identity. He has picked from those he has witnessed and experienced in others in order to organize a composite identity that represents how he would like to be perceived in the professional world. He attempts to validate the characteristics he has chosen.

Cognitively, the resident expands on what he perceives to be optimal knowledge about patient evaluation and management. He can now independently use his knowledge base to analyze a patient's condition, recognize problems when appropriate, and decide on the most well-informed plan for a patient. Probably no one in the unit has a more current knowledge base than the resident at this stage. He demonstrates that independence in making decisions. He also has independent responsibility for consultative advice and care, although he can still be supervised by a faculty member. The resident prepares for board examinations in his specialty, which usually occur at the conclusion of the training program and which further assist him in integrating a knowledge base.

Technically, the resident continues to hone the procedures he deems important. He becomes more proficient performing procedures such as cardiac resuscitation with complex equipment such as a defibrillator. He demonstrates fine motor skills in such delicate manipulations as a lumbar puncture. He is so competent that he can now direct and supervise others on the health team, such as pharmacists, respiratory therapists, and nurse practitioners, in performing the procedures involved in the care of patients. He can evaluate and comment constructively on the results of their work according to specified criteria.

Attitudinally, the resident deals with his own fears and anxieties about the care he provides by demonstrating a calm, outwardly in-control manner. Some residents have learned to express their feelings of frustration, anger, or helplessness openly, while others hide their feelings by not discussing or by merely intellectualizing them. The resident is now committed to the attitudes and values he has acquired, such as being honest with patients, showing individual concern for and to each patient, dealing with noncompliant patients and "crocks," preferring various types of patients, and expressing an emotional detachment and self-esteem. Specific ethics have also been developed and are demonstrated by the resident. For example, the resident treats patient information confidentially, is able to decide which patients should have access to which types of care, respects informed consent, and has viewpoints on treating death and dying. He is able to articulate and discuss personal attitudes and ethics, although he may not choose to do so because of norms prevailing in the educational program.

Psychosocially the resident interacts more confidently and firmly with patients. The resident is more able to accept, be patient with, and persuade patients to accept or help with various treatment modalities he has prescribed or recommended. He demonstrates that "tender loving care," reassurance, and emotional support can be effectively communicated to patients in ways that help patients feel better or adjust to serious conditions. The resident's role as a leader on the ward or clinical team is reinforced as he provides consultations for the team. He now directs the technicians and other health professionals who assist in patient care. He must now discuss patient conditions—with referring physicians if he is in the specialty units of a teaching hospital, or with the physician to whom he is referring a patient if he is in a primary care center. He is now much more sensitive to the quality of his interpersonal relationships and their impact on the successful performance of his responsibilities.

The resident's socialization continues as he takes the next step in the career ladder by preparing for and passing certification examinations, documenting that he has obtained a specific level of knowledge. He is also able to demonstrate his knowledge by spending a significant amount of time as a consultant in either the technical role of a subspecialist or the more general role of a primary care physician. Often the resident in a university hospital will undertake or participate in a small research project that helps him to better understand academic medicine. He is considered a junior colleague by the faculty and often begins to attend professional meetings off campus. He has made a significant commitment to the profession, exudes self-confidence, and now feels like a "physician."

As a learner, the resident has become sophisticated. He can demonstrate ability in life-long learning by being able to identify a particular learning need he may have, by pursuing some deeper concept as a remedy for that need, by organizing his information base with a computer or a reprint file, and by determining when he has completed his task. He has consolidated his knowledge base into a useful structure that will facilitate the way he addresses challenges faced with his patients. He should now be able to function as an independent learner.

The resident at this stage often has a teaching role that is more ambitious than the roles of residents in earlier stages. He is constantly viewed as a role model for the practices, values, and subtleties of the profession. He participates in department conferences, presents topics and cases at seminars, brings new knowledge to bear by active participation in conferences, prepares topics for morning report, reviews individual patient care stages by asking questions and making comments, and structures the activities and assignments of other residents by arranging schedules. He is truly a veteran in the program, with a consolidated, if generalized, knowledge base, who can make a significant contribution to the learning of others.

GUIDELINES FOR FACILITATING RESIDENTS' DEVELOPMENT AS TEACHERS

A resident's development as a teacher of less mature learners in clinical settings depends on the creation of experiences that start where the resident is in his development and stimulate growth to the next stage. This means that a resident's teaching responsibilities should be increased to the level of the resident's competence. The following guidelines are intended to assist in development of a resident's teaching skills.

1. Learning new approaches to teaching, coupled with increasing a resident's responsibility in patient care, can be traumatic or at least unsettling. A resident needs personal support available as he makes those changes. Perhaps a senior member of the faculty can serve as a mentor to one or more residents. Difficult teaching encounters, problem learners, and experimentation with new ideas, new methods, and new responsibilities can be discussed individually. Similarly, the resident may need social support from a group setting in which problems can be presented and discussed. Residents could meet periodically in morning report and, in seminar fashion, discuss teaching as the topic. Change can be painful and, therefore, support mechanisms can be critical in a resident's adjustment and development.
2. Residents who express desire and interest should be assigned significant teaching responsibilities. Not every resident wants to be a teacher and not every resident will be the type of role model who can positively influence younger and less mature learners. Therefore, a systematic procedure should be used to select those teaching residents who are most willing and who have potential. Then they should be assigned responsibilities of which they are capable, but which may be new and more complex than those responsibilities previously accomplished. They should be encouraged to experiment with roles that they have not yet assumed. For example, the resident who has demonstrated a competent bedside teaching style with third-year medical students might be asked to try a different style in a small-group or seminar setting. The systematic assignment of new and different teaching responsibilities can stimulate growth.
3. New roles and responsibilities must challenge the resident but must also be within his reach. If the stage of the resident and the complexity of the responsibility are not taken into consideration, the experience can be harmful. For example, residents at modest conceptual levels may have difficulty implementing a complex clinical evaluation scheme for more than one medical student at a time. Challenge the residents, but do not overdo it.
4. A resident must be provided an opportunity for feedback and for some type of reflection on his teaching. A resident should be helped to develop skill in questioning himself and in examining his own teaching from a variety of viewpoints. Most will not do

this unless they are guided systematically through structured interactions with more experienced clinical teachers. For example, discussions promoting reflection can occur in structured conferences between the attending physician and a resident about teaching assignments. The attending physician can start the discussion by asking the resident how he would analyze his own performance according to a previously agreed-on list of criteria. Such reflection and continual self-analysis, coupled with the actual experience, facilitates growth.

5. The balance between the conduct of teaching and time given to relating that teaching to the principles of teaching and learning is important. The integration of concrete experience with abstract concepts is critical if objective generalizations are to be made and residents are to learn from their experience. For example, a seminar scheduled weekly, in which residents with similar teaching responsibilities gather to discuss their teaching in a manner similar to morning report, can be productive. An attending physician or educator can provide the structure by raising questions that relate the experience being cited to a principle. To support a balance between experience and integration, one study of teaching showed that 3 hours teaching time per week was as effective as 12 hours in influencing growth of the teacher if a weekly seminar was provided to process the experience (Sprinthall and Thies-Sprinthall, 1983). A balance between the two is essential.
6. A teaching development and improvement program for residents should take place over an extended period. A 2-hour seminar, a 1-day workshop, or a statement by the chairman during orientation will not facilitate skill development or movement from stage to stage. Those activities may be sufficient to sensitize residents to the need for change, but they will not facilitate that change. An extended program is crucial. For example, a resident could be asked to videotape a teaching session with a student each month and then to review it with other residents, an attending physician, or an educator. The development of the resident as a teacher should not be organized or viewed as a one-time project; rather, it should be an integral component of an ongoing process of problem-solving and program improvement.

SUMMARY

This chapter has endeavored to present the case for and outline of a developmental approach to the professional development of an individual medical resident. The framework is intended to provide a theoretical basis for understanding the process of a resident's growth. It is not intended to suggest that all residents will achieve all dimensions in all stages, but it is intended to suggest that a resident's developmental stage is related to a qualitatively different level of behavior in performing complex tasks. It is likely that the chapters to come can stimulate developmental growth along the lines described in this chapter. If one knows what the course of development is or should be, then it may be possible to know what responsibilities can be assigned and what educational programs are appropriate at what levels.

PART II

Techniques for Teaching and Evaluating

CHAPTER 3

Our Physician Forebear Sir William Osler as Teacher to Emulate

JAMES A. KNIGHT

When our physician forebear Sir William Osler (1849–1919) was asked what his most important contribution to medicine was, Osler stated simply: "I desire no other epitaph . . . than the statement that I taught medical students on the wards, as I regard this as by far the most useful and important work I have been called upon to do" (Osler, 1905). In using the term *student,* Osler generally was referring to all trainees in medicine—interns and residents as well as students. They were all his junior colleagues, as he described them.

Osler blended effectively student and residency teaching on the hospital wards. He was familiar with the English system of clinical clerks and surgical dressers, a method of bedside clinical teaching, and referred to this system as the source of his inspiration for introducing the clinical clerkships at Johns Hopkins Medical School (Osler, 1945, pp. 318–325). To this, Osler added the German residency system for graduate physicians and the use of hospital laboratories for teaching and diagnostic purposes, thereby creating the most effective system of clinical instruction ever known in America (Ludmerer, 1985, p. 61). Osler emphasized that his method of teaching was not the ward class, in which a few cases were demonstrated, but that his approach was *ward-work,* where the students, interns, residents, and attending physicians all did their share of the work of the hospital. At times, the terms "house pupil," "intern," and "resident" were used interchangeably to describe the medical school graduate who received intensive, clinical training at the bedside in the endeavor that Osler described as ward-work.

During Osler's years at Hopkins (1889–1905), residency training was being developed similar to that conducted today. As Osler resident Campbell Howard reported, the medical residency provided the opportunity for "The Chief" to tutor neophytes in the art, skills, science, and general humanities related to medicine. Along with caring for patients and working in the clinical laboratories, Osler urged and stimulated the residents to study and to write (Howard, 1983).

CHARACTERISTICS OF A TEACHER

Osler's influence on students was profound, and many of the great physicians in American medicine acknowledged this influence. Physicians such as Wilder Penfield, Campbell Howard, Maude Abbott, William S. Thayer, Harvey Cushing, Emile Holman, and Wilbert C. Davison, among many others, spoke often of their debt to Osler. A large company of these accomplished students effectively changed the face of North American medicine during the first half of this century, and their influence continues to this day. In Osler's students one can see incarnate something of the essence of their teacher (McGovern, 1985). He was the acknowledged master teacher of his generation.

One of these students, Harvey Cushing, began working closely with Osler when Osler was professor of medicine at Hopkins and Cushing was William Halsted's assistant resident in surgery. Cushing often referred to Osler's profound influence on him, ranging from Osler's guidance in writing for publication to the acquisition of a library, both current and historical. For example, an early recollection of Cushing was how Osler had kindly admonished him not to neglect to mention juniors connected with recorded cases when Cushing was a young surgical house officer at Hopkins and first trying his "feeble literary wings" (Barondess, 1985). Osler taught by being a great model for Cushing and the other house officers. Osler touched many aspects of their growth and development and could be quite direct in his guidance or counsel, as Cushing's recollections show. Osler had a strong orientation toward young colleagues, and with them his charismatic effect was greatest.

In his book *The Art of Teaching,* Gilbert Highet (1950), in discussing nineteenth and early twentieth century teachers, wrote that the good teachers liked most of their students and most of the rest of the world, and showed it. He went on to say that teachers like Osler "were jolly high-spirited fellows, always cracking jokes and bringing students out as the sun brings out zinnias." Osler's proudest honor was the unwritten title of "student's friend."

Osler spared no effort in preparing himself for his students. Dr. Emile Holman (1969), a former student, remembers him as, "Delightfully informal, erudite beyond comparison, entertaining but surprisingly effective, Sir William Osler enjoyed teaching. So interestingly and compactly were his presentations arranged, it took little effort to remember them."

Even in Osler's day, the phenomenal strides in every branch of scientific medicine tended to overload it with detail. Osler identified the task of the teacher as the winnowing of the wheat from the chaff and in preparing the material in a digestible form. Osler stated further that devotion to a subject coupled with enthusiasm and energy enabled a teacher to keep abreast of new developments but, at the same time, could lead the teacher into pedagogic excesses. Osler spoke of the Reverend John Ward, Vicar of Stratford-on-Avon, who, shortly after Shakespeare's day, made a classification of doctors that has since become well known: "first those that can talk but doe nothing; secondly, some that can doe but not talk; third, some that can both doe and talk; fourthly, some that can neither doe nor talk—and these get most monie." Osler himself classified professors into four groups. First, there is the person who can think but has neither tongue nor technique. A second type is the phonographic professor who can talk but who can neither think nor work. A third is the person who has technique but who can neither think nor talk. The fourth type is the professor who can do all three—think, talk, and work. As with most teachers, ideal and not so ideal, Osler was deeply concerned with what kind of balance should be maintained between the didactic or theoretical and the practical "hands-on" learning in doing. While acknowledging the hospital and the laboratory as the proper place for most teaching, Osler emphasized that the old-fashioned lecture had its place and, although railed against, it should not be eliminated, for there would always be teachers who could present a subject in a more lucid and attractive manner than could be given in a book (Osler, 1899).

In writings that discuss educational or teaching approaches, the argument is often between the right methods or the right teachers, and which approach is more fruitful in attaining one's goal. D.C. Sinclair (1953), writing in *Lancet,* speaks on behalf of the teacher and states that when good teachers and good students are brought together the product will also be good. Osler would surely have met Sinclair's description of a good teacher, but the method or approach in teaching was also of major concern to Osler. The teacher as model was for Osler almost inseparable from the method. While he was acutely conscious of communicating to the student a sense of enthusiasm, a devotion to knowledge, a zest for learning "why," and a compassion in the care of patients, he was also acutely conscious of the teacher as model. Osler emphasized this in a letter to one of his former residents, C.N.B. Camac (1906), in granting him permission to bring together in a book selected passages from Osler's published writings. The letter began with these words: "In the teacher I have always valued the message of the life above the message of the pen." Possibly Osler was saying that there must be no contradiction between precept and practice, no discordant note between the message and the messenger, or else the goal will not be reached.

Osler was a person of many talents, and his skills in teaching, in the care of patients, in writing, and in radiating a genuine humanity have left a mark on medicine that time will never erase. As Stewart G. Wolf has said, although Osler had gained prominence as a pathologist in his earlier professional years, he was first and last a bedside clinician and teacher (McGovern and Roland, 1969, pp. 53–57).

The bedside of the patient became for Osler, early in his career, the setting for his finest teaching. Here his two loves met in a unique fashion—his clinical care of patients and the teaching of his "junior colleagues." Osler summarized the real problem facing medical teachers as "not so much what to teach, but how to teach . . . and how the practical shall take the place of didactic teaching" (Osler, 1899). Further, the practical setting in which he liked to teach offered the opportunity to teach his trainees how to acquire knowledge. In a sense, the sick patient became the medium for teaching and furnished the trainee the medium through which knowledge was obtained. Thus, how to teach and how to learn met in the patient.

RELATING TO STUDENTS

When Osler addressed students, he used the words "fellow students." With such a salutation, a sense of community was formed immediately with those who searched with him into the mysteries of health and disease. Brown has expressed well the charismatic and continuing influence of Osler on his students:

> The more we learned, the more wonderful his boundless knowledge seemed; the wider our vision, the more limitless his appeared. . . . Be-

> cause of him our lives have been better, our successes more real, our failures less hard to bear, for through the tangled skein that spells life each of us knows that in him he has, and will always have, a teacher, a friend, and a true fellow student to the end of the chapter. (Brown, 1920)

Osler saw no appreciable interval between the teacher and the one being taught, only that one was a little more advanced than the other. In such a learning atmosphere, Osler contended that a student would then feel that he had joined a family whose honor was his honor and whose welfare was his own (Osler, 1945, p. 400). Further, Osler believed that every student or trainee, at whatever rank, should be involved in teaching. This, of course, lessened the distance between professor and student and made family membership more of a reality (Osler, 1911a).

Students and trainees in the hospital setting attest to how Osler in working with them acted as a fellow student in guiding them in the examination of the patient, causing them to see what they had not previously noted, and demonstrating how findings should be carefully and clearly recorded (Steiner, 1935).

Further, in these encounters with students, Osler had a way of helping the student present himself in a good light. For example, E.H. Richardson, a former student of Osler and later professor of gynecology at Hopkins, tells of presenting cases to Osler in conferences in the hospital amphitheater. Although one would anticipate with dread a devastating barrage of questions that would serve only to humiliate the student and reveal the student's meager knowledge, this never happened with Osler. Instead, in presenting to Osler, the student gradually relaxed and confidence returned under the hypnotic warmth and glow of a profoundly sympathetic counselor who could be relied on to exhibit the student only in a positive manner that strengthened the student's self-esteem (Richardson, 1959, p. 114).

Osler made education relevant for his students or trainees by integrating compassionate study and informed conduct, by demonstrating a care and concern for what they could become, and by giving them a profound motivation for learning—the hope of becoming better persons. He brought them together through the genius of his friendship and by the way in which he lived his ideals and induced others to share these ideals with him. In his teaching, care of patients, writings, and entertainment in his home, those in training always occupied a place of honor and royal friendship. Osler said repeatedly that students were the inspiration of his life. His ability to inform, instruct, and inspire them was conveyed by both the spoken and written word.

INDEPENDENCE OF LEARNERS

He encouraged his students in their studies to ask "What do I need to know?" and not "What do you want me to know?" He coveted for the students not the role of a puppet in the hands of others but rather a self-relying and reflecting human being. The proliferation of examinations and rigid scheduling of all of the student's time offended Osler's educational sense.

Osler's educational philosophy was built on learning by doing, as self-education under guidance. He taught how to acquire and interpret information. His students and house officers would never see their education as complete, but rather that they must go on studying and investigating as long as they lived. Medical knowledge was not something that was fixed, but something that grew and evolved and was ever changing through the onslaught of new information. When contradicted by empirical discoveries, traditional medical concepts are to be abandoned. Thus, old "truths" could and should be challenged. Knowledge gained by doing and experiencing was to be valued more highly than that learned from traditional authorities, such as lectures and textbooks. "The whole art of medicine is in observation," Osler wrote, "to educate the eye to see, the ear to hear, and the finger to feel" (1945, p. 315). Further, the acquisition of principles should take precedence over the acquisition of facts, for the principles would become the doctor's road map, as well as helping discern between essentials and non-essentials, between wheat and chaff (Osler, 1899). Such an educational approach, according to Osler, helps the doctors in caring for patients to avoid "the-nickel-in-the slot" attitude of mind that has been the curse of the physician in the treatment of disease (Osler, 1905).

A major segment of Osler's life was his constant preoccupation with what we now call continuing medical education (Houle, 1969). Throughout one's life the doctor must genuinely believe that one's education "is not a college course, not a medical course, but a life course, for which the work of a few years under teachers is but a preparation" (Osler, 1945, p. 400).

Osler urged each of his trainees to keep records consistently of his observations and to reflect on them. He urged the carrying of a small notebook that fits into one's pocket and never to ask a patient a question without notebook and pencil in hand. After the examination of a patient, 2 minutes will suffice to record the essentials in the daily progress of the patient. "Routine and system," admonished Osler, "when once made a habit, facilitate work, and the busier you are the more time you will have to make observations after examining a patient" (1945, p.

412). Osler urged the study of the notes taken on one's cases, observing rhythms and consistencies, looking deeply into puzzling observations, and seeing whether a group of cases teaches more than any single case. Through such an approach one could gain wisdom through experience. Only by collecting data and using them could one have sense or wisdom in treating one's patients. Osler made a distinction between knowledge and wisdom and never tired of quoting Cowper:

> Knowledge and wisdom, far from being one,
> Have oft-times no connexion. Knowledge dwells
> In heads replete with thoughts of other men;
> Wisdom in minds attentive to their own.
> Knowledge is proud that he has learned so much;
> Wisdom is humble that he knows no more.

In his teaching, Osler did not hesitate to confront his students. Osler liked the face-to-face relationships with students and demonstrated his concern for them both by support and judgment. He accepted the basic precept that it is the students who must do the learning and that true learning begins with not knowing the answer. Any student in hospital rounds with Osler who dropped a name such as Graves, Laennec, or Von Basedow, after whom diseases were named, was sure to be asked about the person named and not infrequently assigned the task of writing a brief paper on the person and his work (Bean, 1985; Pratt, 1949; Rogers, 1974).

BEDSIDE TEACHING

Osler had a deep interest in medical pedagogy and often commented on the ingredients for good teaching and a good teacher. He suggested a school of medical pedagogy in which able young persons aspiring to the position of teacher could be taught proper methods (Osler, 1907). Moreover, he encouraged his medical colleagues to be interested in becoming successful teachers and pointed out the rewards of teaching in spite of the allure and competition of other activities, such as medical research. At the opening of the new Pathological Institute of the Royal Infirmary in Glasgow he emphasized that point:

> In the hurly-burly of today, when the competition is so keen, and there are so many seeking the bubble reputation at the eyepiece and the test-tube, it is well for young men to remember that no bubble is so iridescent or floats longer than that blown by the successful teacher. A man who is

> not fond of students and who does not suffer their foibles gladly, misses the greatest zest in life; and the teacher who wraps himself in the cloak of his researches, and lives apart from the bright spirits of the coming generation is very apt to find his garment the shirt of Nessus. (1911b)

Osler was imaginative and innovative in his teaching. He made of the hospital a college and did his finest teaching there. He insisted that the wards be thrown open to students. He assigned his students to the wards and remained there with them. Bedside teaching represented a radically different method of pedagogy to what had been practiced in most medical training centers in the United States up to that time. Dr. Hezekiah Saiki of Kyoto, Japan, told of being a house officer with Osler in Philadelphia from 1885 to 1888. He said that Osler spent most of his time at the Blockley Hospital with students and house officers, using his methods of careful history taking, painstaking physical examination, systematic recording of progress notes, the regular use of the laboratory in the study of the patient, and the introduction of students and house officers into the wards and outpatient departments (Davison, 1973). In such a learning milieu, the role of the trainee changed from passive observer to that of active participant in the learning process.

Under the clerkship system, trainees would become an active part of the hospital machinery by spending most of their time on the hospital wards carrying out duties related to their patients' care. Osler noted that all other forms of clinical instruction, including the systematic lecture, the amphitheater clinic, ward or dispensary classes, were but "bastard substitutes" for a system that makes the medical student help in the hospital as part of its human machinery (1945, p. 389).

One of Osler's former students states that after a lapse of 52 years, his recollection of Osler is just as vivid as if he had but momentarily emerged from one of Osler's unforgettable hospital clinics or ward rounds. In describing ward rounds with Osler, this student reveals Osler as master teacher and what was to this student "the personification of the ideal professor":

> At ward rounds, as Dr. Osler moved from one patient to another and sat in turn by the bedside of each one, he listened attentively while the responsible student presented a synopsis of the history, a summary of his examination and ventured a diagnosis. Then, "the Chief," as he was affectionately called, with a bedside manner that I have never seen equaled in dignity, simplicity, and reassurance to the patient, would proceed with his own examination, during which he utilized with exceptional skill as perfectly fashioned and capable a pair of hands as I have ever seen

> possessed by any man. Next, after resuming his seat, he would analyze the story and findings with astonishing brevity and clarity, discarding unessentials, and reconstructing the pattern of the disease under consideration with such faultless logic and precision that each and every such presentation provided his listeners with a word picture that was well-nigh unforgettable. If time permitted, he rarely failed further to adorn these clinical gems with their appropriate historical setting, paying worthy tribute to those by whose labors our knowledge of each specific malady had been enriched, and frequently concluded by casually assigning one or more of the most conspicuous original contributions, often available only in French or German, to the clinical clerk for a synoptic review to be presented at ward rounds one week hence. (Richardson, 1959, p. 106)

Osler emphasized the blending of the old art of medicine with the new science. In this commitment, he had a worthy example in a famous predecessor about whom he often spoke—Herman Boerhaave. When Boerhaave joined the faculty of the medical school in Leyden in 1693, medical practice throughout the world was chaotic and confused by new concepts of chemistry, physics, anatomy, and pathology. Boerhaave organized, distilled, and delivered the useful information from all the rapidly accumulating scientific knowledge of his day and balanced and mixed it with the ancient and traditional art of medicine. Rather than lecture on theory alone, he showed students and his colleagues what to do at the bedside of sick patients. He selected what was useful from an almost overwhelming mass of discovery and rejected an even greater mass of nonsense that was masquerading as discovery (Cushing, 1940). Osler surpassed Boerhaave in separating sense from nonsense by giving the world a book, *The Principles and Practice of Medicine* (Osler, 1892), which remained the pattern of textbooks of internal medicine for a half century. Both Boerhaave and Osler chose the most illuminating setting available for their teaching—the bedside of the patient.

CONCERN FOR AND RELATING TO PATIENTS

Treating and learning were never separated in the care of patients. Osler taught that the doctor must focus on each patient as both a problem of treatment and an exercise in learning. The doctor also would grow and actually be renewed in observing and caring for the sick and the broken. Osler described the interaction with patients in these words: "Amid an eternal heritage of sorrow and suffering our work is laid, and this eternal note of sadness would be insupportable if the daily tragedies were not relieved by the spectacle of the heroism and devotion displayed by the actors." Osler went on to say that nothing sustains you more potently than to recognize in your work the true poetry of life—the poetry of the commonplace, of the ordinary man, of the toil-worn woman, with their loves and their joys, their sorrows and their griefs. And he spoke of the comedy of life spread before doctor and patient and their ability to laugh together at this comedy (1945, pp. 404–405).

Osler's sense of humanity shone in the care of the patients. He inspired his students to emulate him in his care of the lowly and downtrodden. He seemed to be guided by two great Biblical admonitions: "Thou shalt love thy neighbor as thyself" and "Whatsoever ye would that others should do to you, do ye even so to them." Osler urged his students never to forget the rights of patients or their needs. A.D. Gardner recalls one of Osler's clinical lectures to junior students at the Radcliffe Infirmary in which he mentioned, "In my behavior to my patients I make no difference whatever between the high and the low, between a duchess and a cook." Gardner comments that in England, at that time, there was a considerable difference between cooks and duchesses, and most people were inclined to treat them quite differently. Osler's principle in practice struck the students as excitingly enlightened and humane. His radiant humanity emerged as a source of extraordinary clinical success (Gardner, 1969).

A psychological dimension or awareness was very much a part of Osler's bedside care and teaching. Instinctively he knew the right phrase, reassuring gesture, look, or gentle touch. He used suggestion, and he emphasized the therapeutic value of large measures of hope, merrily quoting a Philadelphia colleague who once jokingly defined Osler's practice at the Johns Hopkins Hospital as a "mixture of hope and nux vomica," adding that "the grain of truth in this statement lies in the fact that with many hospital patients once we gain their confidence and inspire them with hope the battle is won" (Osler, 1909).

In the teaching and patient care situation at the bedside, Osler has described what should be there in the person of the doctor: *imperturbability*. Osler defined imperturbability as "coolness and presence of mind under all circumstances, calmness amid storm, clearness of judgment in moments of grave peril, immobility, impassiveness . . . " (1945, pp. 3–4). A patient has described what was there and how profoundly the patient was touched: "In a room full of discordant elements he entered and saw only his patient and only his patient's greatest need, and instantly the atmosphere was charged with kindly vitality, everyone felt that the situation was under control, and all were attention. . . . The moment Sir William gave you was yours . . . with the easy sweep of a great artist's line, beginning in your necessity and ending in your necessity, the precious moment was yours, becoming wholly and entirely a part of the fabric of your life" (Cushing, 1940, 1, pp. 420–421).

ECONOMY OF WORDS

Osler practiced a reasonable economy of words, especially in his teaching. Students marveled at the clarity and preciseness of his words on hospital rounds and in case conferences. In developing such a skill, Osler may well have learned something from an older medical colleague who once confronted him. Osler remembered the experience and liked to tell others about it in order to illustrate the virtues of brevity, relevance, and appropriateness in the use of language. In his early days in Montreal, Osler was called in consultation by an older physician for whom he had done autopsies. It may well have been the first time he had acted as a consultant, and he was pleased indeed with the opportunity. After the examination, Osler was asked to speak to the family. This he did, detailing at great length the symptomatology, diagnosis, and prognosis of the case. After they had left the patient's house, the old doctor turned to him and said, "Young man, you talk too much. For forty years I have practiced medicine with only a nod of the head" (Pratt, 1949).

Another area in which Osler practiced great economy of words was in his letters. He was usually brief but enormously informative and to the point. His humanity, however, managed to shine through these words in spite of their brevity.

PRIORITIES AND PASSIONS

There were priorities and passions in the life of Osler, and most of these had a profound relevance in his teaching and in the educational development of the students, interns, and residents around him.

Osler had the rare ability to place priorities in a proper order. He had such a remarkable sense of what is important and what should be emphasized that many of his judgments have stood the test of time. As Martin Cummings has noted, "With the exception of areas such as clinical therapeutics, which change rapidly, his philosophic and educational views are strengthened rather than weakened by the passage of time" (McGovern and Roland, 1969).

Osler had strong reservations about full-time clinical professors, out of fear that these physicians would become cut off from the way medicine was practiced in the community outside of the university hospital. They then would be less effective in training their students and resident assistants for the real world of medical practice. He advocated strong ties with the medical practitioners who served the public at large in a "ministry of health." He also advocated that each professor be involved in the practice of medicine both inside and outside of the hospital. He knew that the research laboratory could be seductive for full-time professors and that before long there would evolve a set of "clinical prigs, the boundary of whose horizon would be the laboratory, and whose only interest was research, forgetful of the wider claims of a clinical professor as a trainer of the young, a leader in the multiform activities of the profession, an interpreter of science to one's generation, and a counselor in public and in private of the people" (Osler, 1962).

One of Osler's strongest dislikes was the practice of frequent examinations for students, instead of an occasional one. He was convinced that examinations quenched the all-precious investigating spirit of students and made the end and object of study the meeting of certain tests. The examinations were not tests of the capacity to do or to think but how far the student had made himself a phonograph or monotype on which an examiner might play (1907). Osler felt that there were methods more effective and more personal than the written examination in assessing student progress, and he strongly recommended and used other methods in evaluating the level of competence of those in training with him.

Living in "day-tight compartments" represented a philosophy of life of which Osler spoke to students and practitioners alike. He had made the discovery of day-tight compartments early in his life and urged it as a way to prevent what we would today call "burnout." A sentence he had discovered in one of Carlyle's essays made a lasting impression on him: "Our duty is not to see what lies dimly at a distance, but to do what lies clearly at hand." Let the day's work suffice with no thought of tomorrow, for absorption in the duties and tasks of the hour is in itself the best guarantee of ultimate success, he proclaimed repeatedly. In his famous Yale address of April 20, 1913, "A Way of Life," he offered this counsel: "The load of tomorrow, added to that of yesterday, carried today makes the strongest falter. Shut off the future as tightly as the past. . . . The life of the present, of today, lived earnestly, intently . . . is the only insurance for the future. Let the limit of your horizon be a twenty-four hour circle" (1969, pp. 19–20).

The speed and proliferation today of new developments in scientific medicine tax the physician in keeping abreast of these changes. Would Osler's style of teaching and practice have led him quickly to be out-of-date? Not at all! Osler was a fine example of how one should enter the profession only when well prepared, and that preparation must be continued throughout life. From his early years in medicine to old age, in practice as in precept, he bore witness to the physician's urgent need to continue to learn. It represented no idle use of words when at the age of 63 he began an address before the student body at Yale with the words, "Fellow students." Continuing education represented a high priority for him, and at every opportunity he tried to point out to students and colleagues the necessity of this approach in medicine. The central focus of medical education as Osler shaped and reshaped it in his four professorships (McGill, Pennsylvania, Hopkins, and Oxford) was that from the beginning the physician must consider study a lifelong task. He frequently pointed to examples of the consequences of doctors in general practice, in specialty consulting, and in teaching who had failed to improve themselves, to keep up with new advances. He emphasized that medical professors themselves were not immune to a relentless intellectual staleness. In reviewing a medical textbook, Osler pointed out that the book illustrated the difficulty a teacher has in escaping from the bonds in which a routine course, delivered year after year, tends to encircle the teacher with the thoughts and professional opinions of 30 years ago.

Osler felt that doctors in training and in practice should spend some time each day, if only a half hour, in reading great literature. He urged the starting of a bedside library. He emphasized that a liberal education could be had at only a slight cost of time and money. Rest not satisfied only with professional training, he urged, but try to get the education of a scholar. He proposed a way to work toward scholarly development: a half hour of reading each night before going to sleep and in the morning having a book open on one's dressing table. Long before the present-day stressing of the humanitics in medicine, Osler was guiding those around him in the marriage of literature and medicine. Among his many recommendations of what to read were the works of two great physician-writers, Sir Thomas Browne and Oliver Wendell Holmes. Osler described the love of his life as given equally to books and to people (1945, pp. 204–205, 366–368).

Students like to see in their teachers an emotional and intellectual commitment to something so strong that it resembles an addictive passion. Osler had several addictive passions, and two of these he shared generously with his young associates and students: his passion for medical history and his love of great books. He blended these two passions and integrated them creatively in his medical teaching and practice. In a dedicatory address given for a new building of the Boston Medical Library, he spoke these memorable words: "To study the phenomena of disease without books is to sail an uncharted sea, while to study books without patients is not to go to sea at all" (1901). As for medical history and Osler's search through the literature of the past, he sought to offer his students an encounter with their ancestors whose experiences, hopes, achievements, and mistakes had made the human condition what it was. The path of our medical practice is illumined, he taught, by our standing on the shoulders of the doctors who have gone before us. At a time when medical knowledge and practice were changing almost daily, Osler manifested his reverence for the profession by his fascination with the history of medicine. He could caution doctors about how much remained to be learned, and this served as a useful check to the ebullient overconfidence of some of the medical scientists.

CONCLUSION

One can ask how Osler would fare in our era of scientific medicine and high technology. If he were alive today, would machines separate him from both patients and students? Would machines and other symbols of high technology change or distort the bedside setting where Osler did his finest teaching? Probably not, because of the way he embraced and integrated the scientific medicine of his day while maintaining the clinical acumen and spiritual and methodological values of an earlier era of great clinicians. It has been said that Osler was not unlike Henry Ford, Thomas Edison, Alexander Graham Bell, Luther Burbank, and other popular heroes of the early twentieth century who represented and retained "old-fashioned values" even as they forged a technological society (Ludmerer, 1985, p. 135). Thus, Osler today would not let machines distance him from patients or students. His humanistic values would have kept him focused on patient and student, with high technology being always his servant and never his master. For Osler, medicine existed truly as medicine only when the science, technology, and craftsmanship of the physician were practiced with the deepest respect for the humanity of the patient.

With the new science in medicine ascending strongly, Osler recognized and taught that it did not encompass all critical aspects of diagnosis and treatment. There was much that was unique about each person's illness, and that uniqueness could be learned best by nontechnological inquiries based mainly on dialogue. Illness, among other things, was an experience by a patient that invested the illness with meaning. Thus, the doctor had to ask, "What does this illness tell us about this patient and about the family and community from which the patient comes?" A therapeutic regimen would be successful only to the extent that it would meet the needs of the disease as well as the needs of the patient, who modified and felt the effects of the disease in a unique and individual way. Thus, Osler frequently stressed that it was as important to know as much about the person who had the disease as it was to know about the disease that had the person.

The misuse of technology leads medicine to become more institutionalized and its delivery depersonalized and exorbitantly expensive. Yet it must be remembered that doctors practice medicine the way they are taught. Whether doctors retain the personal and humanistic touch and carry this into their practice after they complete their training depends very much on the quality of their training. Osler's ideals of medical education permeated his life and work. These ideals are even more important today and have the capacity to influence profoundly the practice of medicine in spite of a technologically dominated medicine. Osler was one among a few of his physician associates who spent his career preaching and teaching that medical education should have a procedural rather than a substantive emphasis, thereby producing physicians who are thinkers rather than memorizers (Ludmerer, 1985, p. 280). Thinking physicians, as Osler perceived the term, are the ones who in the practice of medicine ask not "What is there to do?" but "Should it be done?" They realize that many techniques and procedures have limited applicability and that in most cases the most reliable information is still obtained from the patient. They are not deluded into believing that they have mastered technology because they are using it. On the other hand, they use fewer tests and procedures because they understand the uses and limitations of technology and are not seduced or mastered by it. Critical thinking, in the way Osler taught and demonstrated it, offers for us today the way to keep science and technology in the servant role. Thus, Osler's teaching techniques and ideals are as relevant today as in his time, and probably even more needed, although no easier to impart.

CHAPTER 4
Clinical Teaching Techniques for Residents

JANINE C. EDWARDS
ROBERT L. MARIER

This chapter presents techniques that medical residents can use when teaching students in inpatient and outpatient clinical settings. These techniques may be useful in other settings and to other teachers as well, although we are addressing residents here.

These techniques can be applied without special equipment, elaborate organizational structures, or support personnel. Many of these techniques are basic and may be obvious to some experienced clinical teachers (Table 4.1).

A brief review of the sources for deriving clinical teaching techniques and the learning process is presented first as background information. This is followed by a discussion of specific techniques.

SOURCES OF INFORMATION

Knowledge of resident teaching can be generated from four sources: (1) research studies, particularly direct observations; (2) perceptions of students, attending physicians, and residents themselves; (3) experts' opinions; and (4) adaptations of social science (particularly education

TABLE 4.1 Clinical Teaching Techniques for Residents

- Plan ahead
  - Hold work rounds early
  - Make a work list
  - Group and divide the tasks for maximum efficiency
  - Meet with team at end of day to plan the next day
- Win cooperation by teaching
- Tell students to ask for help when they need it
- Communicate objectives and evaluation criteria
- Use patients for teaching whenever possible
- Think aloud
- Build knowledge base
  - Associate ideas
  - Organize ideas
  - Encourage reading
  - Ask questions and explain
    - Rephrase or simplify questions
    - Address questions first to the student responsible for the patient
    - Wait for student to think
    - Consider the setting: patient present or not
    - Select an appropriate questioning style during case presentations
    - Use strategy of open-closed-open questions to discuss cases
- Set a good example
- Motivate learning
  - Appeal to current and future interests
    - Place student in role of practicing physician
    - Remind student to prepare broadly, regardless of specialty interest
    - Remind student of course requirements
  - Arouse conflicting thoughts
  - Attribute success to efforts, and failure to lack of effort
  - Display high expectations
  - Emphasize each learner's improvement rather than competition
- Give feedback
- Evaluate performance
  - Find out evaluation responsibilities
  - Write evaluation notes periodically
  - Advise attending physician of problem students
  - Fulfill due-process requirements
  - Evaluate attainment of the objectives
- Problem-solving strategies
  - Have students *independently* gather patient data and formulate the differential diagnosis
  - Pose hypothetical cases
  - Use a "data-respository" for group problem-solving
  - Study decision analysis
- Teaching procedural skills
  - Explain the procedure
  - Demonstrate the procedure
  - Provide supervised practice

and psychology) theory and research. Material for this chapter has been drawn from all four sources.

Little information has been gathered about resident teaching from research studies; some studies of attending physician teaching, however, can be applied to resident teaching. Payson and Barchas (1965) observed attending teaching rounds and resident work rounds. They described significant differences of time spent talking about physical factors, psychosocial factors, and theory. Medio et al. (Chapter 13) have also studied resident work rounds, while others have studied attending rounds (Adams et al., 1964; Mattern et al., 1983; Maxwell et al., 1983; Reichsman et al., 1964; and Weinholtz, 1983). An observational study by Bosk, a sociologist, (1979) gives an insightful view of the resident culture. Weinholtz describes in detail an observational study that, if conducted, would yield much valuable information about resident teaching (Chapter 8).

Perceptions of clinical teaching are a second source of information. Two surveys of resident teaching time have been published. Brown (1970) determined that house staff spend approximately 20% to 25% of their average work week supervising, teaching, and evaluating others. Two thirds of the residents indicated they would like training in teaching skills. Barrow (1966) surveyed second- , third- , and fourth-year medical students, who indicated they received approximately 31% of their learning from residents and interns.

Expert opinion is a third source. Experts could be residents, clinical faculty members, or others. The opinions of the authors, an experienced clinician and an educational researcher, are given in this chapter, as well as those of others. The fourth source is theories, research findings, and practical experience about learning and teaching from education and psychology. Large bodies of knowledge from these disciplines can be adapted to clinical teaching by persons familiar with the system of physician training. The monograph "Effective Clinical Teaching" by Stritter and Flair (1980) is an example of this approach.

INFORMATION-PROCESSING MODEL OF MEMORY

The goal of teaching is to promote learning. Hence, teaching techniques should support and cultivate learning. Clinical teachers must understand the essentials of the process that goes on in the learner's mind. For that purpose, a brief explanation of the learning process is given here.

During the past twenty years, research in cognitive psychology has sought to discover the structures and processes of human memory.

Today, human memory is thought of as an information-processing system composed of three structures: a sensory register, a short-term memory, and a long-term memory.

Information is represented in short-term memory in two forms: verbal and visual (analog, spatial). In long-term memory, information is certainly represented in verbal form. Whether or not visual images are represented in long-term memory in spatial (analog) form is a matter of controversy. The weight of recent research evidence, however, suggests that visual images are stored in long-term memory (Klatzky, 1980; Kosslyn, 1980). Because clinical teaching centers around patients, visual images are important in physicians' thinking.

Long-term memory is thought to be a vast network of two types of knowledge. Following Steward and Feltovich (Chapter 1), we refer to these as *knowledge base* and *problem-solving*. Knowledge base refers to the store of verbal information; knowledge about facts and things. Problem-solving is knowledge about how to perform cognitive activities. Procedural skills are frequently included in the category of problem-solving (procedural knowledge) (Anderson, 1985), but to avoid confusion among medical educators, we will describe the teaching of procedural skills separately.

Knowledge is widely believed to exist in the form of logical propositions, which represent meaning in an abstract manner without preserving exact wording. A proposition is the smallest unit of knowledge about which a true or false judgement can be made (Anderson, 1985). An example of a proposition is "Heart failure causes pulmonary congestion because left ventricular filling pressure rises." Figure 4.1 is a model of the long-term memory network.

SPECIFIC TEACHING TECHNIQUES

Plan Ahead

The resident in charge of the service has a broad set of responsibilities. He is responsible for overall management of patients, setting priorities, and making adjustments as needed under the broad direction of an attending physician. He must assess the performance of subordinates and assign work appropriately. He must keep track of everything, doing whatever is needed to ensure timely evaluation and treatment of the patients. He must keep his attending (staff) physicians apprised of major developments/questions. On top of all this, he must teach.

Efficient utilization of time and resources is essential—not only for patient care, but also for teaching. If the team is poorly managed, im-

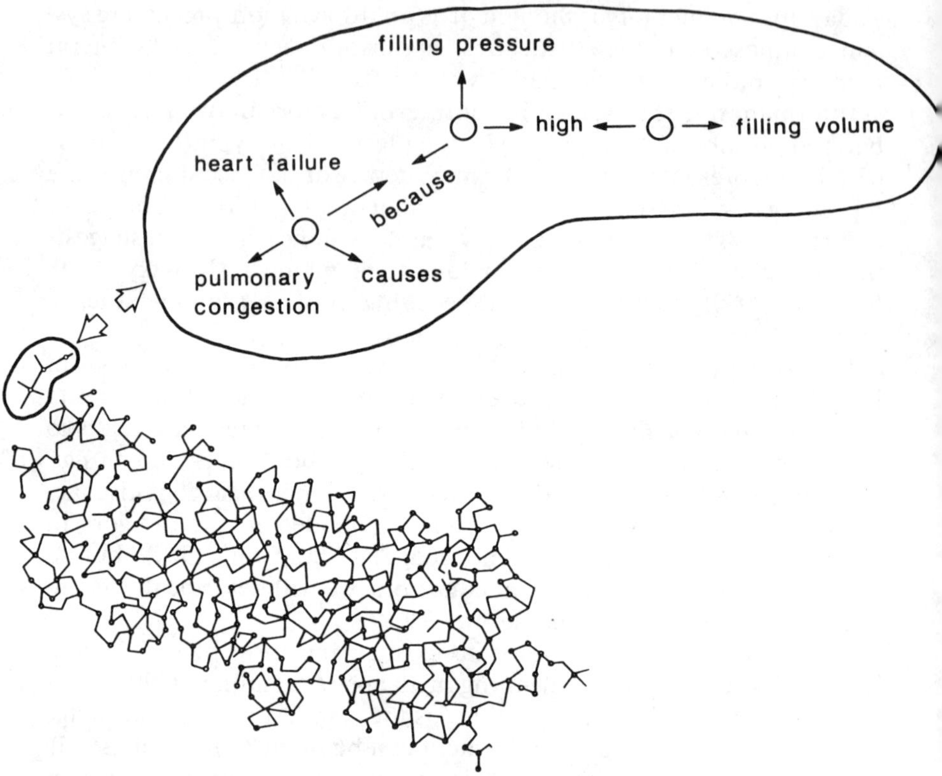

FIGURE 4.1 The propositional network. Each proposition is linked to other propositions through common ideas.

Adapted from Ellen D. Gagné, *The Cognitive Psychology of School Learning*. Copyright © 1985 by Ellen D. Gagné. Reprinted by permission of Little, Brown and Company.

portant tasks are deferred or forgotten. Some members of the team are busy while others are not. There may be a shared feeling of wheel-spinning and frustration. There may be little time for teaching.

All aspects of a clinical rotation will work more smoothly if residents use some specific management and communication techniques during the first 2 or 3 days. These include establishing work routines and duties, telling students to ask for help if they need it, and orienting students to the objectives and evaluation.

The work day should be carefully organized. Work rounds should be held early with clear division of labor. A work list is helpful and can be used during the day to keep track of things. Tasks should be grouped and delegated for maximum efficiency. The team should meet at the end of the day to plan for the next day.

At the beginning of the rotation, the resident should orient team members to the objectives and tell them how their work will be evaluated. He should explain the duties, and he should also establish a work routine, because this makes the work go efficiently and allows time along the way for teaching and learning. Efficient managing facilitates both patient care and teaching.

Win Cooperation

Good residents quickly discover that teaching helps them win the cooperation of students. Students are much more willing to help out with the work if they are given something in return. As a general rule, they will follow the resident around willingly and help out as a member of the team when they perceive that they are appreciated and treated as learners as well as workers. Students should be told that the only serious mistake they can make is not asking for help.

Communicate Objectives

Communicating objectives (learning outcomes) is basic to any teaching relationship. In the beginning, the teacher must make sure that the learner knows what is expected. This makes learning more efficient and evaluation more equitable (Popham, 1973).

Residents should find out from clerkship directors what the objectives are for students so that they can reinforce and facilitate their attainment. Moreover, they must tell the students and interns what is expected of them in the day-to-day routines.

> *Example*: A student is called on to present a case at morning report. He starts off well enough but gets bogged down: "This 57-year-old male is admitted to the west service with a chief complaint of cough and sputum production. He has a complicated medical history with diabetes, congestive heart failure, and cirrhosis." The student then goes into great detail about the patient's past history and is interrupted by the chief resident who tells him to come to the point: "What are you doing? We have 10 patients to cover in the next 30 minutes. Just tell us why the patient came to the hospital this time."

The student should have been told how to present a patient in morning report.

Use Patients

Residents should use patients for teaching whenever possible. Patients make lasting impressions on students and the basis for this may relate to how the mind stores information—as charged images.

It seems logical for physicians to think about disease processes in images because the human body is a physical, concrete object existing in space. Organs are located in spatial relation to other organs and to the skeletal-muscular system. Physiological functions occur in space encapsulated by the body. The patient's body, then, is an image that assists in encoding information. Abstract concepts learned from textbooks become concrete and meaningful when related to a human whose body gives physical evidence of disease signs and symptoms.

Medical students should generate increasingly more elaborate mental images as they progress from textbook learning in the basic sciences into clerkship experiences with patients. Ingenious experiments have demonstrated that people do amalgamate images to generate new ones (Kosslyn, 1980).

Affect, or emotion, associated with the patient charges the image, helping to fix it in memory and making it easier to retrieve. The learning atmosphere with a patient present is charged with emotion. All the reasons which brought the student to that point—concern for the sick patient, the intellectual stimulation of solving a problem, the sense of performing a duty, even the necessity of presenting the case to others—serve to fix the experience in the student's memory.

Yates (1966) recalls that Giordano Bruno summed up these thoughts well: "Images must be lovely, active, striking, charged with emotional affects so that they may push through the doors of the storehouse of memory" (p. 294).

Think Aloud

Residents can teach many things to students by "thinking aloud" as they go about their daily tasks of patient-care. This flow of thoughts put into words for the student's benefit is a way to explain and demonstrate. Making covert thoughts overt reveals the learning process in action. Thinking aloud is an important technique for teaching problem-solving and procedural skills.

Build Knowledge Base

Increasing knowledge is a basic learning task. This can be accomplished by associating and organizing ideas, encouraging reading, and questioning and explaining.

Associate Ideas

A major principle is that one learns by associating propositions (Wittrock, 1986). Students increase their knowledge base by relating new information to it. By relating learning to other patients, facts (diseases, treatments, anatomy, pathophysiology), or structure (categories), the student sees interrelationships and hooks new information onto a growing network of information.

> *Example*: A ward team is discussing a patient with diabetes. The resident asks a student, "Why does this patient have diarrhea?" The student hesitates. The resident asks what organs are affected in diabetes mellitus. The student indicates that the kidney, eyes, and blood vessels are involved. Another student suggests that the nerves are also involved. The resident points out that the gastrointestinal tract should be added to the list and explains the reason for this. He has hooked a new piece of information to the students' growing knowledge of diabetes.

Organize Knowledge

Teachers can facilitate knowledge retrieval from long-term memory by helping learners organize their knowledge. Steward and Feltovich (Chapter 1, p. 7) explain the differences in expert and novice problem-solving strategies. The expert has more knowledge pertinent to a given problem area, and that knowledge is more highly organized. He has more connections for each proposition and his entire knowledge base is organized hierarchically (Gagne, 1985; Feltovich, 1981). It is important for teachers to assist learners to organize their existing knowledge and integrate new knowledge.

> *Example*: A student has presented a patient with fever of unknown origin (FUO) to the senior resident on the service. The resident asks "What is the differential diagnosis of fever?" The student begins a jumbled list of diseases that might produce this symptom. The resident interrupts, "Let's approach this more systematically. What are the major categories of disease that produce prolonged fever?" The student says that infection, neoplasia, connective tissue disease, and a miscellaneous group are the major categories. The resident says, "Right. Now let's consider each category, and list the most common causes of fever in that category. When we have finished, we will go back and see how this case fits in."

Encourage Reading

Osler (1901) said that to care for patients without books to guide is to sail on unchartered waters. Patient-centered reading helps to increase and particularly to organize students' knowledge base about specific medical problems. General medical reading, of course, is beneficial, but patient-centered reading has this advantage: the student is highly motivated to learn about a particular problem by his responsibility to care for the patient. Students and residents often complain about lack of time for reading. Time shortages are a part of professional life, however, and students must be taught to use prudently whatever time they have. Patient-centered reading allows students to teach themselves throughout their careers.

Students should be given a list of recommended texts and strongly encouraged to use one of these as a basic resource, reading and rereading main sections. Current journals should be consulted for highly specialized problems. Students should be encouraged to learn how to use the library efficiently to find information. They should be encouraged to share some of what they have found with the group, sometimes in the form of summaries or note cards or reprints. This gives all students an opportunity to demonstrate their own commitment to the group learning process.

Ask Questions

Questions serve two purposes: to stimulate knowledge and to guide problem-solving. Teachers should show students how to answer questions by helping them search through their own knowledge base, relating new information to what they already know, estimating probability, sorting or refining concepts. Questioning is frequently more valuable to the learner than explaining because questions require the learner to recall what he already knows, make associations within the memory network, and apply that knowledge. Explaining is useful when the learner has not yet acquired knowledge or cannot apply knowledge to a particular problem.

Many classification schemes or taxonomies of questions have been proposed and applied to teaching (Foley and Smilansky, 1980; Graesser and Black, 1985; Hyman, 1979). Weinholtz (1983) categorizes questions according to type (probing, clarifying, or mixed) and frequency (high, medium, or low). The advantages and disadvantages of using different questioning styles during case presentations are presented in Table 4.2. The use of a particular questioning style should depend upon the student's ability and experience, as well as on the complexity of the case. Weinholtz considers the medium-frequency mixed style most advantageous because the instructor can assess the student's knowledge and presenting skill without disorienting him. This style is the most difficult to use, however.

One frequently used distinction is between open and closed questions. Closed questions are narrow and designed to elicit knowledge. Open questions require problem-solving. An example of a closed ques-

TABLE 4.2 Advantages and Disadvantages of Different Questioning Styles

Questioning style	Advantages	Disadvantages
High-frequency probing	Provokes student into preparing presentations carefully	Flusters and disorients student, thereby inhibiting instructor's ability to assess depth of knowledge and presenting skill Prolongs presentations and rounds
Medium-frequency mixed	Enables instructor to assess depth of student's knowledge and presenting ability Provokes student to prepare carefully, while stimulating interest	Most difficult approach to implement, because optimal number of probing questions is hard to gauge
Low-frequency mixed	Enables instructor to assess very selectively depth of student knowledge, while providing very clear indication of presenting skill Easy approach to implement	If left unguided, the student may ramble, consume time, and bore other team members
Low-frequency clarifying	Provides clearest indicator of student's ability to present a case Most preferred by students	If left unguided, the student may ramble, consume time, and bore other team members Instructor must take notes or concentrate very carefully to remember follow-up questions

From Donn Weinholtz, Directing Medical Student Case Presentations, *Medical Education,* 1983, *17,* p. 367.

tion is: What is the patient's temperature? An open question is: What are the causes of fever? In some cases the teacher may just want to know specific bits of information. If time allows and the setting is appropriate, the teacher should go beyond closed questions.

Other questioning techniques include rephrasing or simplifying a question. Clinical teachers should allow students thinking time; they should be careful not to answer their own questions. We think that questions should be addressed to one student (the one responsible for the patient), at least initially. Finally, the setting should be considered (Weinholtz, 1983). Some questioning can take place in the patient's presence, but the patient must be included in some way—e.g., by defining terms and explaining the significance of what is being said. Very detailed or critical questions should be addressed away from the patient.

Here is a general questioning strategy for discussing a patient case with one student. The student presents the chief complaint, history, and physical findings according to the prescribed format. Then the teacher begins the discussion with an open question such as "What is your impression?" This question allows the student to reason as far as he is able without guidance. Only when the student falters or is wrong does the teacher move in with closed questions dealing with specific facts of pathophysiology and etiology. These closed questions probe the student's knowledge base and stimulate him to relate clinical findings to textbook knowledge. When the teacher has guided the student through the line of reasoning to the most basic concepts, the questions can begin to widen out into more open questions allowing the student to generalize to principles and to related cases. This strategy can be diagrammed as two pyramids, apexes touching (Figure 4.2).

The following example illustrates good questioning and explaining techniques.

Example: A surgical team is called to the Accident Room to assist in the care of a patient who has been run over by a truck. Once the patient is stabilized, the resident turns to a student and says, "What is the first thing you have to do for a patient like this?" The student hesitates. The resident prompts, "Do you have a list in mind? You know, A, B, C. I am referring to general principles now". The student says, "Initial steps include stopping hemorrhage and immobilizing the fractures." The resident explains that the airway must be secured and circulation reestablishied first. Then he goes on to describe a short protocol for managing major trauma cases. Finally, the resident asks, "What do you think will happen to this patient?"

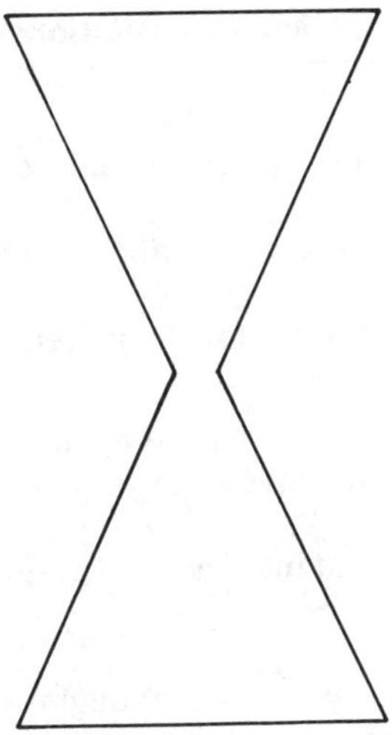

FIGURE 4.2 A questioning strategy for discussing patient cases with one student.

We have organized major points about questioning as well as other teaching techniques into a concise Checklist for Teaching Case Presentations (Table 4.3). Residents may find it useful to look at the checklist from time to time as they work with students. It may also be used to review videotaped teaching performance.

Set a Good Example

People learn from observation (Bandura, 1977). In a very real sense, each teacher is a reflection of his own teachers and the ones before them. Teachers are constantly modeling—correctly or not—what they themselves have seen or want to be. Residents model not only the science of medicine, but also the art. Students learn how to interact with patients and with other physicians from residents. Students must see honesty, diligence, and selflessness as the basis for all else in medical practice. They must see skilled physicians at work examining, operating, thinking, comforting, teaching, and doing all the other things that are the content of medical practice. Negative examples set by residents and attending physicians can decrease students' dedication to duty and foster cynicism.

Live role models may be supplemented with historical models. Osler, who is the physician–teacher role model par excellence (Chapter 3), spoke about this very well.

TABLE 4.3 Checklist for Teaching Case Presentations

I. To communicate objectives

1. Ask or tell the student what information should be included in the presentation before starting.
2. Ask or tell the student how the case presentation should be organized before starting.
3. In general, establish the ground rules for the presentation.

II. To question

4. Question (rather than lecture) to stimulate student's thinking.
5. Ask closed questions to probe student's knowledge of patient case and medical information.
6. Ask open questions to help student integrate and evaluate information and plan treatment.
7. Phrase questions clearly.
8. Wait adequate time for student to organize thoughts and respond.
9. Avoid unnecessary and frequent interruptions.

III. To synthesize information and analyze the case

10. Provide or elicit medical knowledge relevant to case (such as pathophysiological principles, pathogenesis, risk factors).
11. Assist student to organize or summarize presentation, focusing on important facts.

    Establish with student a concise, organized problem list.
12. Direct student in clear and organized line(s) of reasoning to obtain a diagnosis.
13. Review pertinent facts in relation to the diagnosis and discuss their significance and implications.
14. Pose hypothetical situations to expand and deepen student's understanding.

IV. To provide feedback

15. Comment on *specific* positive and negative points.
16. Recommend improvements.
17. Be objective so that the student does not feel he is being personally attacked.

V. To consider generalities

18. Demonstrate support, understanding, and encouragement of student (good eye contact, attentive body posture).
19. Acknowledge limitations of one's own knowledge.
20. Encourage use of medical literature and other medical personnel to aid in problem-solving.
21. Take notes or use chalkboard, if appropriate

> This higher education so much needed today is not given in the schools, is not to be bought in the market place, but it has to be wrought out in each one of us for himself; it is the silent influence of character on character and in no way more potently then in the contemplation of the lives of the great and good of the past, in no way more than in the touch divine of noble natures gone. (Osler, 1901, p. 61)

Osler set the example in his own life of how to relate to students. He considered students his "junior colleagues" and addressed them as "fellow students." He put no distance between himself and students, but instead tried to make students feel as members of a family to bring out the best in each (Chapter 3, pp. 38–39). Being a living example is perhaps the best way to motivate learners.

Motivate Learners

Motivation is the process of initiating activity (Wittrock, 1986). Residents can motivate others to learn in several ways (Table 4.4). One way is to appeal to the current and future interests of learners. Put the student in the role of a practicing physician. Ask him to develop a plan or write orders for an actual or hypothetical patient.

Examples

1. A 23-year-old woman in the third trimester of pregnancy presents to the Emergency Room with vaginal bleeding. The chief resident is called to see the patient. He asks a student "Should we admit the patient?" The student responds, "Well, the differential diagnosis includes. . . . ," the resident repeats his question, the student tries to dodge the question again, but the resident won't let him get by and says, "Put yourself in my place. There are reasons for and against admitting this patient, but you have to decide now." Eventually the student says "I would admit her." The resident says, "Good, now let's move on to the next patient." The student realizes perhaps for the first time that he is called to a life of action and must be prepared.

TABLE 4.4 Techniques to Motivate Learners

Appeal to current and future interests
Place student in role of practicing physician
Remind student to prepare broadly regardless of specialty interest
Remind student of course requirements
Arouse conflicting thoughts
Attribute success to effort, and failure to lack of effort
Display high expectations
Emphasize each learner's improvement rather than competition

2. The ward team arrives in the X-ray Department. The resident turns to a student and says. "You have shown an interest in x-rays. You will be the radiologist this afternoon. Are you up to it?" The student who plans to go into radiology has his big chance!

These approaches appeal to the student's interests. Other interests might include their own hobbies, their families, or medical problems they have observed in their own families or among friends. Such personal information can be gained during coffee breaks, lunches, and socializing after-work hours. An alert teacher uses all this information to motivate learners.

A different approach may well be needed for students showing little interest in the subject matter and who are planning to specialize in other areas. Some residents may be able to use case material to illustrate basic science points that students might need. Students may need to be alerted to changing technology and practice and the importance of being broadly prepared for this. In extreme cases, a resident may need to point out that before they can do whatever they are planning to do, students have to pass the present course, and the requirements are to do this or that.

Thoughts can motivate actions. Conflicting thoughts raise cognitive dissonance, which gives rise to motivation for finding the facts or the truth, thereby resolving the dissonance. One way to arouse conflicting thoughts is to ask questions instead of making statements, or to present conflicting information or opinions (Gagne, 1985). Sylvius, a famous seventeenth century clinical teacher, liked to provoke disagreement because he believed that intellectual dissension resulted in consensus of opinion and improved morale; it also enabled him to express his own opinion (Linfors and Neelon, 1980). Care must be taken not to make such conflicting thoughts threatening to the learner, however. Making an intellectual game out of conflicting thoughts and playing the devil's advocate reduces the sense of threat. Knowing when and how to motivate a particular student or resident requires judgment. Most intelligent and willing students will profit from challenging exchanges. Sensitivity to the learner's ability and degree of motivation, however, is required.

Attributions of success or failure can motivate, if used properly. If students think that success is due to effort and they see themselves as hard-working, they are more likely to persist longer in learning and achieving. Likewise, if students think that failure is due to lack of effort, they may try harder. On the other hand, if students think that failure is due to bad luck or circumstances beyond their control, they are likely to be less motivated (Weiner, 1980).

Teacher behavior and affect can heighten motivation. If the learner thinks that he has control over his own actions, he is likely to put forth greater effort. Teachers who display higher expectations for students and who respond with anger rather than sympathy over poor performance can motivate students. Displaying sympathy for failure implies that the learner has no control over the learning situation (Gagne, 1985).

Emphasizing the individual's improvement rather than competition among persons can lead to increased effort and achievement (Gagne, 1985). Residents should be careful about pitting one student or intern against another in a spirit of playful competition. Rather, improvement over previous performance should be emphasized with each individual.

In summary, the following motivational techniques have been described: appeal to the current and future interests of learners; remind students to prepare broadly regardless of their specialty interests; remind students of course requirements; stimulate conflicting thoughts; attribute success to effort and failure to lack of effort, if this is feasible; set high expectations; and emphasize each individual's improvement.

Give Feedback

Feedback takes place when a person is offered insight into what he actually did and the consequences of that action. Medical students often complain that they receive little or no feedback to guide them. Residents can change the atmosphere of clinical education by giving feedback to the students. Feedback can reinforce correct learning and prevent recurring mistakes, as behavioral psychology has amply demonstrated (Biehler, 1978).

The following guidelines are recommended (Ende, 1983): (1) give feedback frequently and as soon as possible; (2) use first-hand observation; (3) make feedback specific; (4) make feedback descriptive and informative, not judgmental.

Mistakes, widely recognized to be part of the learning process, must, of course, be corrected. Before criticizing a student, however, consider whether or not the student should be expected to know the answer. Consider also the type of mistake—intellectual versus normative, repetitive, or attitudinal. Also consider the setting (bedside, corridor, or private conference room). Sharply critical feedback—especially that dealing with overall performance—should be given in private, in most cases. It should *never* be given in front of patients.

Students become more knowledgeable and skilled if they receive feedback regularly. They are grateful to residents who give feedback and usually cooperate better in working with these residents.

Feedback should be based on first-hand observation, if possible. Residents may be in a better position than attending physicians to give feedback to students relating to many of the routines of clinical work.

Specific detailed information helps the person to see himself objectively. What some might consider "general feedback" is merely a performance rating which usually cannot guide future learning. Telling a student, "You did all right" after he has spent an hour examining a patient may increase his confidence, but it does not help him improve his physical examination skills. Commenting on the particulars of that performance will help more; for example, "You should ask more specific questions" or "You might find it easier to have the patient sit on the edge of the bed for this purpose".

As a general rule, feedback should not judge or evaluate the learner's intentions. It should be descriptive. Descriptions are limited to what was said and done or how it was accomplished. For example, "You appeared to be upset in that patient encounter. Why were you upset?" The teacher might then go on to talk about how to deal with feelings in patient encounters, how to use feelings as a signal. "After all, you are responding to something." Feedback that implies judgment or evaluation of a person's motivation or values which are personal may make students defensive. Nonetheless, feedback like this must be given in some cases—but it should be done away from others, if possible. In most situations the feedback person must be perceived as an ally of the learner, not as a judge. A relationship of basic trust must exist between the resident and the student.

Evaluate Performance

Residents are frequently asked to give an opinion of students, formally or informally, at the end of a rotation. This duty may be imposed without advance notice. To avoid any such surprises, residents should find out at the beginning of each rotation what, if any, evaluations are expected. The resident should be alert throughout the rotation to each student's progress. Periodic notes about performance will make the final evaluation more detailed and balanced.

Another aspect of the relationship between resident and student relates to the student functioning as a member of a service unit. He must be held accountable by his superordinates. Residents should question students in order to determine if they are doing their job. Before students have earned the trust of residents, questioning can be intense with complete accounting of every action demanded. Is the student meeting basic expectations? Is he "on top of the situation"? If he is, the questions may shift from what to why, and the resident may lead the student through a reasoning process.

Students (or residents) may make two types of errors (Bosk, 1979). Errors of the first type are technical or judgmental and are seen as part of the learning process. This type of mistake relates to a lack of experience or knowledge. The second type of mistake is normative and is seen as a basic defect. This type of mistake relates to a lack of diligence or honesty and includes failing to disclose problems fully and honestly, missing important findings, quarreling with other health care personnel or failing to secure cooperation of patients and their families. Generally, normative errors are not tolerated. The amount of a resident's monitoring is inversely related to his assessment of a subordinate's competence (Bosk, 1979).

Mistakes are missed by residents for various reasons. Rotations may be short. Because of the corporate aspect of clinical work, those who know what is going on rescue those who do not. Questions may be directed at a group rather than at individuals. This limits, and may preclude, competent assessment of that individual's performance.

Judgments about attitudes and interpersonal skills are often difficult to make. These should be assessed as specifically as possible, but sometimes a resident just has a "gut feeling" about a student. Student absence from required functions is usually a symptom of more serious problems. Whenever problems arise, the resident should alert the attending physician immediately and document in writing the specific problems.

Frequently students having serious problems slip through the evaluation system because nobody recognizes the problems in time to do anything about them. Due process requirements must be met. The requirements for due process are: (1) inform the student of the objectives; (2) present him with a written notice as a warning of failure; (3) provide time and resources to the student so that he may correct the deficiency; (4) provide an appeal system.

At the time of final evaluation, the resident should evaluate the student in terms of objectives set forth at the beginning of the rotation. Residents should be able to evaluate students' skill in taking histories, performing physical examinations, and performing common procedures. In fact, residents usually have more direct supervision of students' learning in these areas than have attending physicians. Personality factors, of course, indirectly influence the assessment of students' performance, but these should not unduly sway the resident's judgment about student attainment of the objectives. In the final evaluation, if the student has met or surpassed the minimum standard, emphasis should be placed on progress made during the rotation. Table 4.5 summarizes techniques to evaluate performance.

TEACHING PROBLEM-SOLVING STRATEGIES

Research

Problem-solving is an important aspect of medical education to teach. It is also the most difficult. Research on medical problem-solving has been conducted within three paradigms: (1) an information-processing approach describing steps in reasoning; (2) correlational studies of physician performance on various types of problems; (3) the decision-analysis approach, which prescribes algorithms to improve clinical judgment. The information-processing line of research emphasizes the hypothetical-deductive nature of the process (Barrows and Tamblyn, 1980; Elstein et al., 1978; Kassirer and Gorry, 1978). According to this view, the physician perceives initial clues from the patient, generates multiple hypotheses about the nature of the problem, applies an inquiry strategy (questions, physical exam, tests) to refine, rank or eliminate the hypotheses, formulates the problem, and decides on a course of management (Barrows and Tamblyn, 1980). McGuire (1984) raises two questions about this line of research: Are the tasks used in this research really problem-solving? Can the process accurately be termed hypothesis generation? She proposed that pattern recognition, schema recognition, or concept formation, instead of true problem-solving, may be the type of knowledge involved in clinical reasoning.

Research on problem-solving during the past few years has consistently found low correlations between a physician's performance on one problem and performance on a second, dissimilar problem. The low correlations hold for all formats of problems: live simulated patients, paper and pencil patient management problems, and computer simulations. These findings do not support the assumption of a universal problem-solving process. Two implications arise from the

TABLE 4.5 Techniques to Evaluate Performance

Find out evaluation responsibilities
Write evaluation notes periodically
Advise attending physician of problem students
Fulfill due-process requirements
Evaluate attainment of the objectives

findings. Either the measures are unreliable or the clinical problem-solving process varies greatly for a given person (Norman et al., 1985).

Berner (1984) asserts that the assumption of one universal problem-solving process has been proved invalid. She proposes that multi-dimensional categories of problems are necessary for investigation. Her proposal agrees with current findings about the domain specificity of problem-solving in other areas of knowledge (Gagne, 1985). In general, research about problem-solving in medicine and other domains (e.g., physics, geometry, chess) seems to be converging on the following conclusions. Expert problem-solvers are distinguished from nonexperts primarily by their knowledge base rather than by their general problem-solving ability. Experts have more knowledge and better organized knowledge in their specific domain (area of knowledge). They have learned to represent problems in more abstract or general terms to which they can readily predict solutions. They perceive recurring patterns in problems presented to them and associate their solutions to these patterns (Anderson, 1985; Steward and Feltovich, Chapter 1, p. 7; Waldrop, 1984). These conclusions fit well with physicians' perceptions of their own problem-solving ability. A specialist in infectious disease may believe he is expert in that domain, but that he is less expert in kidney disease, for example.

Finally, formal decision analysis in teaching problem-solving must be considered. The algorithms used in all forms of decision analysis are complex; nonetheless they are useful.

Pauker and Kassirer (1980) have developed a method for making management decisions based on the probability of certain outcomes. They have developed algorithms which may be useful where sufficient outcome data exist in making individual decisions. They point to a general strategy that should be part of medical training. The decision-analysis approach has three characteristics: it is explicit, quantitative, and prescriptive (Weinstein and Fineberg, 1980). It is explicit in that the decision maker must analyze the components of the problem and then synthesize them. Mathematical formulas are used to calculate the probabilities and values placed on possible outcomes. This approach is prescriptive, rather than descriptive as is the problem-solving approach. It gives physicians a method for deciding what they should do. Soon, teaching the clinical reasoning process may be facilitated and raised to higher levels of skill through the use of Intelligent Computer Assisted Instruction (ICAI) programs. ICAI programs differ from traditional computerized patient management programs, or computer-assisted instruction (CAI), because they contain expert reasoning strategies (hence, intelligent). The traditional CAI patient simulations contain medical knowledge and a few simple problem-solving strategies, all built into the same program. ICAI contains separate programs for the medical knowledge and problem-solving strategies. The separate program allows expansion of the reasoning strategies and greater flexibility in their use. GUIDON, developed at Stanford University, is an example of an ICAI program. GUIDON can do more than say student answers to questions are right or wrong and branch to further explanation; it can actually reason about the expertise required to solve the problem. ICAI programs simulate the type of discussion students might hold on ward rounds with residents and attendings (Clancey et al, 1984). Future students and residents may use these powerful simulations to form and practice their own clinical reasoning processes as a supplement to experience with live patients and direct encounters with teachers.

Teaching Problem-Solving

The major technique for teaching problem-solving involves demonstrating the reasoning process and providing practice with guidance. This is similar to the technique for teaching procedural skills (see pp. 72–73) (Anderson, 1985).

Residents can demonstrate problem-solving by thinking aloud as they reason out their patients' problems and management. Practice in problem-solving can be provided in several ways.

Residents should arrange periodically for students to interview and examine a patient and formulate a diagnostic impression *without help from charts or other persons*. A resident should observe part or all of this and discuss it with the student. Having to collect the data and figure out the diagnosis and treatment largely on his own is exactly what a practicing physician does. Students will not learn the process adequately if "groupthink" is the only method used to teach problem-solving. Students are quick to recognize and appreciate the learning benefits from such opportunities.

An effective technique is for the teacher to pose case material from his own experience or even hypothetical cases that serve as a framework for teaching. This may be the best way to find out how the student thinks by himself. Prepared cases often reflect the thinking of others who consciously or not may lead the student through the questions or even provide all the answers through discussion or in write-ups that the student may have read.

Many experienced teachers have sets of cases or stories that they use, because these are good examples of important problems. Residents should be encouraged to do the same.

> *Example*: A patient with chronic obstructive lung disease has been admitted to the hospital. Once he has been stabilized, the resident tells the student about another case—a man with much more severe disease who was admitted to the hospital. He provides the student with data on the patient's blood gases and asks how the student would handle the case. He might even give sets of hypothetical values for the blood gases, seeking interpretations of each and asking about treatment plans. He might then tell the student what would happen if his plans had been adopted. The exchanges may be made more realistic by creating time pressures. For example, in the middle of working through one case the resident might tell the student that he has been called to another area of the hospital to evaluate a patient who has developed GI bleeding. At the same time he might refer to the family of the third patient who may be dying and who are asking to speak to him. How would the student deal with all of this?

A technique for teaching problem-solving to a group is described by both Engel (1971) and Kassirer (1983). According to this approach, the student presenter serves as the "resource man" or "data repository." This student takes a proxy role for the patient; no one else in the group has any information about the patient. After the student has given the chief complaint, the teacher invites the team to question the "patient" to procure more data. Each questioner must justify his question in terms of a diagnostic hypothesis or rationale for information that would relate to the diagnosis. If the group agrees with the student questioner, the student data repository responds as is appropriate. The response could be one of relating details about the present illness, past history, physical findings or laboratory results. The resident then asks to explain the data and relate it to his working hypothesis. Requests for information on results of certain tests or treatments can be rejected by the instructor. In more advanced groups, the instructor can move quickly to diagnostic or treatment questions. This method is close to the real life process of clinical reasoning. Each member of the group can take part in the overall reasoning strategy by activating the associated propositions in his particular memory network. All of the intermediate details of the diagnostic process are exposed. Mistakes in the reasoning process can be corrected immediately.

Finally, students should be encouraged to study decision analysis as another way of building problem-solving skills. Many of the variables in a given problem are quantified. Studying decision analysis helps students learn to work with probabilities in problem-solving.

In summary, residents can teach problem-solving in the following ways: (1) think aloud; (2) have students *independently* gather patient data and formulate differential diagnoses; (3) pose cases from previous experience or hypothetical cases; (4) structure team problem-solving with one person as the "data repository"; (5) study decision analysis.

Residents who actively teach clinical reasoning may find it satisfying to know that they are helping students to develop general problem-solving strategies. They are multiplying their effectiveness by teaching others, and their own intellectual power is reproduced and regenerated in the interactive process. This nurturing of brain power is what makes teaching most exhilarating.

PROCEDURAL SKILLS

Research

Teachers are always in the position of being observed or of being demonstrators. This is most obvious when teaching procedural skills. The correct method for examining patients and for carrying out various procedures must be taught by example. Residents are often in the best position to teach these things to students because they spend much time with them at the patient's bedside, in the admitting room, and in other areas where the day to day problems of medical practice are encountered.

Research in educational psychology, military training, physical education, and movement science has demonstrated that procedural skills develop in three stages: the cognitive, the associative, and the autonomous stage. In the cognitive stage, students develop knowledge of the skill. In the associative stage two things happen: errors are gradually eliminated and the knowledge is transformed into procedural skill. The outcome of this stage is successful performance of the skill. In the autonomous stage, with practice over time, the speed and accuracy of the skill increases (Anderson, 1985; Fitts, 1962). Students and interns struggle with stages one and two in learning to perform clinical procedures. Residents develop expertise (the autonomous stage) with simple procedures and struggle with complex procedures.

Teaching Procedural Skills

The technique for teaching procedural skills involves the following components: (1) demonstrate the procedure; (2) verbalize each step of the procedure as it is demonstrated; (3) provide practice; (4) give feedback during practice; the feedback may be verbal and manual.

dent tries it. This is a well-established pattern in training programs. Questions like "Have you seen this done or have you done this before?" come first. There might be related procedures that the student has seen or done that might be helpful. The relationship should be brought out in discussions with the student. The student may have read about a procedure or seen video, slide, or model demonstrations that would have given him visual images and information.

Residents must demonstrate every aspect of the procedure for the student including selecting the best approach, adapting to whatever circumstances exist, and relating to the patient before, during, and after the procedure. This process should be verbalized, if possible, at the time in the presence of the patient. Depending on the type of procedure and the patient's level of consciousness or anxiety, the explanation may have to be given elsewhere.

Residents should point out landmarks and other technical details during demonstrations to help the students associate the visual, aural, or tactile images with whatever else they know. If the patient is awake, the resident should explain things to the patient during the procedure.

Supervised practice is essential to develop expertise in performing skills. If possible, residents should provide practice and supervise students immediately after demonstrating a procedure. They should also give opportunities for repeated practice over a period of time. Artificial models may be used to supplement practice.

Complex skills may be a composite of subskills. If the subskills are independent, they should be identified and taught separately and then practiced as a whole (Fitts, 1962).

A good example of teaching a procedure is provided by Bosk (1979). In this example, the procedure is explained, demonstrated, and practiced. The learner's effort is supported initially by the teacher's hand. The hand is withdrawn by stages as the student learns to operate on his own.

> *Example*: Carl, the intern, was closing an incision while Mark, the chief resident, was assisting. Carl was ill at ease. He turned to Mark and said, "I can't do it!" Mark said, "What do you mean, you can't? Don't you ever say you can't. Of course you can." "No, I just can't seem to get it right." Carl had been forced to put in and remove stitches a number of times, unable to draw the skin closed with the proper tension. Mark replied, "Really, there's nothing to it", and taking Carl's hand in his own, he said, "The trick is to keep the needle at this angle and put the stitch through like this," all the while leading Carl through the task. "Now go on." Mark then let Carl struggle through the rest of the closure on his own.

SUMMARY

Residents are teachers as well as learners, and they can be more effective if they use sound teaching techniques. We have presented specific teaching techniques including the following: plan ahead, win cooperation, communicate objectives, use patients, think aloud, build a knowledge base, set a good example, motivate, give feedback, and evaluate. Techniques for teaching problem-solving and clinical procedures, which are complex skills, have been emphasized.

We are impressed with the abundant talent most residents have for teaching and express our own appreciation to them for teaching us so much about the process.

CHAPTER 5

Developing Lecture Skills

NEAL WHITMAN

I knew a university anesthetist. His lectures put the whole class asleep.

—Anonymous

Residents are often asked to lecture to medical school classes or to talk informally to ward teams. Developing lecture skills during the years of residency training thus becomes a worthy pursuit, particularly inasmuch as most practicing physicians by virtue of their professional status are called upon to speak before clinical and community audiences. Medical students and residents frequently complain about lectures, and deservedly so. Many lectures are boring, befuddling, or time-wasting. Here we show how a person can improve his own lecture skills and can put some punch into lectures.

WHY LECTURE?

In an effort to improve lectures, the In structuional Development Program at Pennsylvania State University printed six frequent complaints in their newsletter (1982):

1. Lecture objectives were unclear.
2. Lecture was disorganized.
3. Lecturer did not relate to students.

4. Lecturer did not respond to students.
5. The lecture was boring.
6. The lecturer did not include opportunities to ask questions.

Each of these complaints deserves a short comment.

1. Often the objectives are unclear to the audience because they are unclear to the lecturer! Effective lecturing begins with the presenter understanding clearly the main points he or she intends to cover. In a manual for the Eastman Kodak Company, Kenny (1982) suggests that the key to success is to set a target and hit it! The target might be thought of as the "big picture," and every lecture should have one. For example, in a presentation to a house staff journal club, a resident might want to highlight clinical situations in which a high positive predictive value or a high negative predictive value is desired. Having this target in mind will guide the presenter as to choice of material, examples, and audience participation.

2. Many lectures are not well organized. Instead, there is an unindexed compendium of facts. A lecture is more effective when it has a definite beginning, middle, and end.

3, 4. Relating and responding to the audience members also is important. The speaker should not bury himself or herself in notes or text. One notable problem arises when the medical lecturer turns off the lights so that slides can be shown. Relating or responding to students in a dark room proves to be difficult. Use of slides will be addressed later in this chapter.

5. Some teachers say that their lectures are boring because the subject is inherently boring. My own view is that there is not a boring subject under the sun. People, not subjects, are boring. The late Jacob Bronowski, noted poet and scientist, argued that no imaginative activity is dull to those willing to reimagine it for themselves (1978). This chapter will explain how to instill that kind of involvement.

6. Finally, students complain when lecturers do not allow time at the end for questions. It can be very frustrating for students to be confused by some point raised by the teacher and not have an opportunity to question the teacher about it. It is more effective to leave time for questions, rather than oblige the audience members to approach the speaker at the front of the lecture room when the lecture is over. At that time, the classroom usually is noisy and chaotic. I suggest leaving at least 10 minutes for a 1-hour lecture and 15 minutes for a 90-minute lecture.

For lectures to be effective, students must know what they are supposed to learn. Thus, a lecturer first must determine what their needs are. Assessing the audience and tailoring the lecture to their needs is critical to being successful. In a clerkship lecture, a resident might want to underscore pathophysiology, whereas in a case conference he might choose to stress patient management issues. When presenting at a continuing medical education course, new approaches to patient management might be emphasized. Everyone is busy, so one should be sure that the lecture is *on target* for the audience.

Without a doubt, the editors of *Change Magazine* were correct in stating in their *Guide to Effective Teaching* (1978): "Nothing is worse than a poor lecture, disorganized and badly delivered." However, they also were correct in adding, "But nothing is more effective than a good lecture, combining substance with showmanship." Residents probably have heard lecturers at their worst and best, the former perhaps more frequently than the latter. Unfortunately, we often "do as we have been done unto." Instead, we should strive to emulate the few exemplary lecturers we have heard. They likely have won teaching awards. They are positive role models and, by following their example, we can learn much about teaching.

In a survey of medical school award winners, Whitan and Ferrey (1986) asked, "To what extent are teachers born or made?" The majority by far responded that they made themselves into good teachers. Although personality may play a role in the success of some of these award-winning teachers, most believe that the basic skills of becoming an effective lecturer can be learned.

According to studies conducted at the State University of New York at Albany and at Rutgers University, when students were asked to describe professors who had done the most to improve their thinking, *least important* were qualities of personality. The five *most important* qualities (McLeish, 1976) were:

1. Systematic organization
2. Ability to encourage thought
3. Ability to explain clearly
4. Enthusiastic attitude toward the subject
5. Expert knowledge

After comprehensively reviewing the research on lectures, McLeish concluded that the lecture is open to serious criticism if used as an all-purpose teaching method (1976). Effective lecturing begins with recognizing what can be accomplished with a lecture. Basically, two objectives can be achieved in a lecture. First, audience members can leave a lecture knowing facts that they did not know before and, second, they can acquire an understanding of the interrelationships and applicability of those facts. In other words, can learners comprehend or grasp the meaning of the material? Note that objectives describe the changes in the learners, not the behaviors of the teacher. Knowing and understanding are examples of *cognitive* objectives, that is, they describe changes that occur in the minds of the learners. According to a taxonomy of cognitive objectives developed by Bloom et al. (1956), *knowledge* and *comprehension* are lowest-level cognitive objectives.

As an example of a knowledge objective, one aim of a lecture to third-year medical students on a medicine clerkship might be for them to be able to recall the ranges of normal vital signs for various adult age groups. This relatively low-level objective might be necessary for students to accomplish a secon aim of the lecture, that they be able to discuss the physiology involved with vital signs, which is an example of a comprehension objective (Inglis and Marazon, 1983).

Higher level objectives are *application* (using the knowledge in new situations), *analysis* (breaking a subject down into its parts), *synthesis* (Putting the parts together in a new way), and *evaluation* (making judgments about the subject). To be realistic, a speaker should not expect learners to achieve these higher level objectives in a lecture. At best, a teacher can model these in a lecture; but for learners to achieve them, more active involvement is needed than is possible.

As an example of higher-level objectives, consider the following objectives written by Inglis and Marazon (1983). Why would students have difficulty achieving from a lecture, and why would they need to be more involved than is possible in a lecture?

Application: The students will be able to integrate vital signs as they relate to myocardial patients being admitted to the ICU.

analysis: The students will be able to interpret the implication of vital signs outside the normal range.

Synthesis: The students will be abel to write management plans based upon the assessment of vital signs, some within normal ranges and others outside the normal range of the MI patient.

Evaluation: Given a patient with an acute MI, the students will be able to develop the problem list, recognize the possible complications, and recommend specific therapeutic measures.

Knowledge and comprehension are interrelated because facts are best learned and remembered when they are known, understood, and have meaning. In a review of the psychological literature, Higbee (1977) found that "One of the determinants of how easy something is to learn is how meaningful it is to the learner. If it doesn't make sense, it will be hard to learn; the more meaningful it is, the easier it will be to learn" (p. 37). The spirit of this "principle of meaningfulness" was captured by the British physicist Ernest Rutherford (1871–1937), who believed that he had not completed a scientific discovery until he was able to explain it to others (Highet, 1950). It is this spirit that lecturers should bring to their material. Some residents might worry that such deliberate emphasis on meaningfulness will lead to underestimating the level of the audience's understanding. However, though this is possible, a review of the research indicates that lectures more often overestimate the level of understanding (Bligh, 1972). One outstanding teacher recommended that instructors "approach and organize their subject as if [the students] know too little about it" (Lowman, 1984, p. 11).

As an example of making a subject meaningful and understandable, Dr. Martin Samuels, associate professor of neurology at Harvard Medical School, delivers a lecture in which he replaces the nebulous category of "cardiovascular accident" with *stroke* (a sudden or rapid onset of a neurological deficit due to vascular disease lasting more than 24 hours), and with *transient ischemic attack* (TIA) (the same as stroke, but lasting less than 24 hours). Furthermore, he breaks down strokes into major categories, ischemic (thrombotic and embolic) and hemorrhagic (hypertensive intracerebral and subarachnoid). The success of his lecture depends largely on Dr. Samuel's ability to make sense, to be organized, and not to go over the heads of his listeners. In the lecture, he presents his personal views of how nuerology should be practiced and, until he writes his own neurology primer, those views cannot be read in a book. A resident should begin the process of developing personal views of medical practice and incorporating these into his lectures. Lectures will be meaningful and understandable when they make sense of complicated subject matter and are organized so that learners can remember it.

Making a subject understandable and meaningful is the *raison d'être* of lectures. After all, most of the facts can be found in books and journals. What a teacher can provide in a lecture that does not appear in print is what one scientist called the "inner relevance" of the material (Kestin, 1970). Similarly, Stanford Ericksen, the noted Michigan educator, emphasized the need to make a subject worth knowing: "Most instruction involves a two part process: presenting information while at the same time indicating its worth" (1980, p. 5). The need to personalize the material was highlighted by a story about the behavioral psychologist B.F. Skinner (1957), who in the 1950's developed "teaching machines" that presented programmed instruction to students. Apparently, when asked if his machine would replace teachers, he replied, "If it can, it should." In other words, human beings deserve to be replaced if they do not do what books or teaching machines cannot do: *be personally responsive to the learners.*

To help personalize the material, Dr. Samuels gives examples in his "Stroke–TIA" lecture that show why being able to classify so-called cardiovascular accidents more specifically makes a difference in treatment, and he provides patient examples to demonstrate each difference. A lecturer's presentation will be more personal when it shows why what is recommended will make a difference and when patient examples are included.

In organizing material for a lecture, residents may wonder how much material to include. In his review of the research on lecturing, Bligh (1972) found that students remember more when told less. Giles et al. (1982) found that the worst recall was for information presented during the first 15 minutes of medical lectures, presumably because additional information presented later in the lecture displaced in memory information presented earlier. Educational psychologists call this "retroactive inhibition," a phenomenon further documented in medical lectures by Russell, Hendricson, Williams, and Herbert (1984), who studied student rentention of information by delivering three versions of a 50-minute lecture on the fibrositis syndrome. In the "low-density" lecture, 50% of the time was devoted to new information, whereas the remaining time was used for explanation and examples. In the "medium-density" lecture, 70% of the time was used to present new information, and, in the "high-density" lecture, 90%. On tests administered immediately after the lecture, as well as 15 days later, students learned and retained information best from the low-density lecture. During what stage of an hour-long lecture are people most alert and most likely to remember the information presented? Conflicting evidence exists. Giles et al. (1982) found that the information presented between the 15tha nd the 30th minutes was remembered best. McLeish (1976), in a review of research on lectures, reports a number of studies that show that efficiency is at a maximum during the first 5-minute "warming up" period. Over the next 40 minutes, student and lecturer efficiencies decline steadily. Then in the last 15 minutes, both lecturer and students climb back up toward a relatively high level of achievement. Although these results from different studies are not entirely congruent, the conclusion can be drawn that listeners' attention is best near the beginning and end of an hour's lecture.

In addition to making the material meaningful, one should organize the subject so that the audience can follow the main points. Unfortunately, some teachers follow the advice given by the King to the White Rabbit:

> The White Rabbit put on his spectacles. "Where shall I begin, please your Majesty?" he asked. "Begin at the beginning" the King said, very gravely, "and go on till you come to the end: then stop." (Lewis Carroll, 1866)

The point is that a lecture should not be one long list of facts. Instead, at the start, the lecturer should let the audience know what the major points will be. Then, each major point can be addressed, followed by a summary. This approach, attributed to U.S. Army trainers, has been described as, *"tell 'em what you're gonna tell 'em; tell 'em; and tell 'em what you told 'em."* In the field of educational psychology, there actually is a basis for this approach, first proosed by D.P. Ausubel (1968), who described the benefits of "advance organizers" that bridge the gap between what learners already know and the new information to be acquired. Providing advance organizers for the audience is like creating files in a new computer program—there must be a place for data to be stored.

As an example of providing an advance organizer, consider a lecture on preconceptual counseling delivered by Dr. Neil Kochenour, associate professor of obstetrics and gynecology, University of Utah School of Medicine. Because this topic is so broad, it is helpful when he tells the audience, "First, I will discuss two maternal diseases which *may adversely affect* pregnancy: diabetes mellitus and phenylketonuria. Then, I will discuss two maternal diseases which *may be adversely* affected by pregnancy: cardiac disease and thromboembolic disease. With all four diseases, I will demonstrate how preconceptual counseling can improve outcome."

In preparing for lectures, residents often ask whether a handout would be helpful. When properly constructed, handouts can be helpful, but if a handout has too much material, it can promote a passive attitude in the learners because "everything they need to know" is there. If a handout has too little material, it likely will be just another piece of paper for students to throw away. I recommend the "partial handout," which includes a lecture outline, some of the important facts, and key tables and figures. In a study of handouts in medical student lectures, Russell et al. (1983) found that the partial handout was a good compromise between comprehensive handouts, which may be valuable for review but encouraged passivity in class, and skeleton handouts, which promoted alertness during the lecture.

ATTRACTING AND MAINTAINING ATTENTION

When planning a lecture, one should consider how to attract and maintain the attention of the audience. Students must become mentally engaged in the lecture material. If learners remain totally passive, little learning will occur in lectures. For new knowledge to be retained and understood, the listeners must think about the material as it is being presented to them. Overcoming the relatively passive role of learners is the major challenge of lecturing (Whitman, 1983). Successful lecturers have a "black bag" of techniques to attract and maintain attention, an *armamentarium,* if you will. One technique to attract attention at the start of the lecture is to tell a relevant anecdote. One of the most successful anecdotes I have heard was told by a physiology teacher trying to get across the point that urine is essentially water and salt present in the body in excess. He told a story about his honeymoon, when he and his wife took a canoe trip in a wilderness area. Because of the hordes of mosquitoes, they did not want to leave their tent at night once they got into it. They wanted to empty their bladders in the tent, but the only available container was their coffee pot. Knowing there was nothing harmful in urine, except perhaps a few bacteria from the urethral orifice that would be killed by boiling, they used their coffee pot at night to empty their bladders and to brew coffee in the morning (Mouw, 1981).

In addition to telling an anecdote, other techniques to heighten attention include posing a dilemma or raising a key issue. The major principle is to pique the curiosity of the audience, to stimulate their interest, keeping them alert enough to want to listen to the rest of the lecture. Using techniques to attract attention provides an opportunity to be creative.

After raising the audience's attention, the next challenge of lecturing is to sustain that alertness. This is not easy, and, in my experience, the biggest problem with medical presentations is the inability of lecturers to keep listeners interested. Maintaining attention is so difficult because, when communication is one-way, the average adult will pay attention for only 15 to 20 minutes, at which time the mind wanders involuntarily. The phenomenon has been well documented in the college teaching research reviewed by Davis and Alexander (1977) and in a study of medical students conducted by Stuart and Rutherford (1978). The reason for this attention loss is clear: Speaking is more active than listening. In a lecture, when learners function only as passive listeners, continuous attentiveness is difficult. Wilbert McKeachie, at the University of Michigan Center for Research on Teaching and Learning, highlighted this problem in realistic terms: "The student in a lecture is usually passive and sometimes asleep—a condition not conducive to maximum learning" (1978, p. 22).

In publishing his observations of the presidential address at the annual meeting of the British Association for the Advancement of Science, H.G. Frost (1967) noted that the president, Lord Brain, while not in the class of Sir John Gielgud, was a good speaker. Nevertheless, his notes at that activity are as follows:

> 9:03 Lord Brain starts.
> 9:12 My attention has wandered. Some people have closed eyes.
> 9:18 About 10 percent in view show signs of attention wandering.
> 9:20 Perhaps one-third of audience is fidgeting.
> 9:28 People looking at their programmes.
> 9:30 Hard to make myself concentrate.
> 9:38 Everyone in sight has now let attention wander.
> 9:42 Whispered conversation on the platform.
> 9:46 Lord Brain refers to world population: general alertness.
> 9:48 Altertness passes.
> 9:49 Lord Brian makes a small joke. Only a feeble titter.
> 9:50 One or two really asleep. One man reads—newspaper I think.
> 9:52 Unless I concentrate, sounds like a stream of platitudes.
> 9:56 End. Applause. (p. 282)

These observations may describe lectures we all have attended—or have delivered. The solution is clear: The one-way communication pattern of "I talk–you listen" has to stop. In other words, every 20 minutes or so a lecturer should use a teaching technique that will provide an opportunity for two-way communication. By occasionally providing a more active role for the learners, the speaker will be able to engage them in the lecture material and maintain their attention.

The black bag of techniques holds five major techniques that will provide a more active role for the audience members: *questioning, brainstorming, demonstrating, role playing,* and *problem-solving.*

Questioning

This technique includes asking questions of the audience and welcoming questions from them. In a large lecture room, it is important that the teacher paraphrase answers to his or her questions and repeat questions from the audience. Audience members become frustrated when they can hear only half of the exchanges between the lecturer and other members of the audience.

When the lecturer asks a question, he should show tolerance for a short delay in awaiting an answer. Research on the behavior of "waiting times" shows that many teachers allow only 1 to 2 seconds before they answer their own questions (Rowe, 1974). Three to 5 seconds may seem like a long time to wait for an answer, but, believe me, it is not a long time for those in the audience to try to think of an appropriate answer. Research also indicates that many teachers allow less than 1 second in responding to an answer. In particular, if the answer is correct, one naturally tends to respond immediately. Waiting for a few seconds, however, provides an opportunity for the respondent to expand on his or her answer and for the rest of the audience to evaluate the answer as well.

In general, the questions asked should be open-ended, that is, have more than one acceptable answer. Such questions maintain attention better than do closed-ended, single-answer questions. Asking only closed-ended questions can turn questioning into quizzing, an activity that can easily turn off an audience. Remember that the major principle is to have audience members feel involved, not sense that they are "on the spot." If, for example, one were lecturing on acute renal failure, asking, "During the diuretic phase, is the risk of periocarditis high or low?" would be closed-ended. It would be more open-ended to ask, "Why would the risk be high or low?"

How those in the audience are called on will depend upon the size and type of audience. In a lecture for medical students, some closed-ended questions might be asked to assess their knowledge level and to get their attention. For example, in a lecture on shoulder pain, one could ask, "What type of tumor is most apt to cause shoulder pain in a 60-year old woman?" In a large group, the speaker might ask for a volunteer, whereas in a small group, he might call a student by name. In a lecture for residents, a participant might be asked to share what he knows about metastatic carcinoma resulting in shoulder pain in a 60-year-old woman.

In asking questions, avoid the "guess-what-I-am-thinking game" in which the lecturer asks what appears to be an open-ended question, but is in fact looking for a particular answer. When this game is played, the teacher rejects what normally would be considered acceptable answers until the "correct" answer is given. This type of questioning can turn off many audience members and is not a good way to maintain attention. If an answer is not "on the mark," one should extrapolate from it whatever is possible with embellishment. You can embellish as necessary to have it be a proper answer.

In addition to asking questions, consider asking for questions. Traditionally, this is done at the end of medical lectures. As a technique to help maintain attention, however, a speaker might want to consider stopping 20 minutes into a lecture and asking, "I have been presenting information that may be new to many of you. At this point, do you have any questions about the material covered so far?" Questions asked by audience members can lead to important clarifications and can help wandering minds refocus on the subject matter. When using this technique, one should remember to repeat each question so that everyone in the audience knows what the question is before they hear an answer. When this technique becomes more comfortable, the speaker might want to invite other audience members to answer the questions as well.

Brainstorming

A special type of questioning is called brainstorming. It is a teaching technique used to generate a variety of creative ideas. In brainstorming, an open-ended question is asked and as many answers elicited as possible. Usually, writing the ansers on a blackboard or flip chart proves helpful. While brainstorming, one should not evaluate the ideas as they are expressed; otherwise the audience members may become inhibited. The major principle is broad participation.

As an example of brainstorming, when lecturing on the epidemiology of tuberculosis a speaker might be making the point that the incidence in the United States has risen recently. A good example of brainstorming would be to ask, "What are the possible explanations for this phenomenon?" Possible responses might include the increase of immigration of refugees from third-world countries, the increase of travel by Americans to third-world countries, the decrease of funding for public health probrams that screen for tuberculosis, the overconfidence by providers that tuberculosis is no longer an important problem and the failure of medical schools to teach this subject anymore. It would be important not to agree or disagree with these responses as they are given. After recording all the possibilities generated by the audience, one then could comment on them, agreeing or disagreeing appropriately.

Demonstrating

A demonstration also can be an excellent way to maintain attention. By using an experiment or some actual performance, a lecturer can bridge the gap between theory and practice. Of course, it is important that the demonstration work; some practice and rehearsal may be necessary. The major principle of this teaching technique is that a memorable learning experience be provided.

An advantage medical lecturers have is the availability of live patients. For most medical students, residents, and clinicians, patient demonstrations are memorable and meaningful. As an example, I gave a physiology lecture on a dare by our Department of Physiology, "The Biologic Mechanisms of Chronic Pain." The faculty in that department were curious to see how an education specialist would present this material. To help maintain attention in the 1-hour lecture, I demonstrated the involvement of cognitive and emotional factors in low-back pain by interviewing a patient in front of the class. I questioned the patient for 10 minutes and offered the students the opportunity to ask questions for another 10 minutes. This patient demonstration occurred midway in the lecture.

By every measure, the lecture was successful. The patient's responses and involvement helped to reinforce some of my main points and to maintain attention. As the lecture ended many students flocked to the front of the room to ask the patientmore questions and to talk with me. They never knew that this lecture was outside of my field of expertise. In contrast to their obvious involvement, the following scenario was observed in another lecture to the same students in the same course:

> The lecture began at 1:00. After 40 minutes of densely presented information, the students were noticeably restless. At 1:50, the teacher said, "We're almost done. Hang in there." The class, scheduled to end at 2:00, ended at 2:10, and the students rushed out of the lecture hall.

Had he used the techniques of questioning, brainstorming, and demonstrating, singly or in combination, that lecturer could have helped maintain the students' interest. I give him credit for recognizing that the students were losing attention. Unfortunately his repertoire of techniques to gain attention apparently was limited to the admonition to "hang in there."

Role Playing

The technique of role playing, although similar to demonstrating, requires audience participation. In role playing, an audience member adopts an assigned role and behaves n ways he or she believes characterizes a particular type of person. Role playing can be an effective lecture technique, for example, in portraying doctor–patient interactions. When using role playing, one must be as specific as possible in assigning roles and describing the situation in which the roles are to be played.

As an example of role playing, Dr. Jerry Klein, then Director of

Adolescent Medicine at the Michael Reese Hospital and Medical Center, Chicago, delivered a lecture on adolescent history-taking to pediatrics residents. Midway in the lecture, he asked one resident to volunteer to take the history of a 15-year old boy who the day before had been sent to the hospital emergency room because he had been acting out violently in school without any apparent provocation. When I walked into the room for the interview, wearing jeans and dangling a cigarette from the corner of my mouth, the class saw at once that I would be role-playing the "student." Dr. Klein had instructed me for my role: be cooperative if the resident did certain things, such as enforce the no-smoking rule (a no-smoking sign was prominent in the room); and be uncooperative if the resident did not establish certain guidelines, for example, that the interview would be confidential. In this instance, the resident provided me with reason to be uncooperative and his history-taking did not go well. Then Dr. Klein continued the lecture, making use of what had occurred in the role play.

When planning a role play, one should determine how long to allow it to continue. Once the role play starts, however, the lecturer should avoid interrupting until its time is up. Then, time for debriefing is allowed, with comments from the role players. Also, the audience members should be asked to comment on their observations. Thus, a role play may require 10 minutes to be played and 10 minutes for debriefing and discussion. Sometimes the audience members may want more time for discussion. because of the time required, a speaker might consider using this technique for lectures that are scheduled for more than an hour.

Problem-Solving

An activity that leads to a value for an unknown, problem-solving usually encompasses both a strategy and elements of skill necessary to carry out the strategy. In the field of medicine, problem-solving usually refers to a hypothesis-driven approach, similar to the hypothetico-deductive reasoning approach attributed to scientists (Amnerican Board of Internal Medicine, 1979). A small but growing store of research data suggests that exposure to a broad repertoire of medical problems is important to the learning of medical problem-solving (Elstein, Shulman, and Sprafka, 1978). In addition, engaging learners in the same process used by clinicians seems to be beneficial (Barrows and Tamblyn 1980).

Thus, besides helping to maintain attention, involvement of medical students and residents in clinical problems during a lecture probably contributes substantially to overall learning. One approach to medical problem-solving, suggested by an internist in the clinical setting, takes this tack: Provide the audience with a patient's age, sex, race, and presenting complaint; then invite the learners to ask for historical physical, and laboratory data aimed at diagnosing and treating the patient's "problem." In this approach audience members must justify their requests for information. For example, the student requesting information might be asked, "What diagnostic possibilities do you have in mind?" or "What do you expect to learn from that?" After the rationale for the question has been given and the lecturer has answered it, he could then ask, "Did that change your thinking?" or "What did you learn from that?" (Kassirer, 1983).

The technique of problem-solving can be used for more than maintaining attention in the middle of a lecture; it can be used as a format for the entire presentation. With a large group, furthermore, the audience can be subdivided into small groups, assigning each a problem to solve with the instruction that they report back to the whole audience in 10 minutes. Each group could work on the same medical problem or on its own specific problem. Successful use of the problem-solving technique in lectures necessitates that the problems be selected with care. Criteria to keep in mind include problem frequency, urgency, and mismanagement.The point is to select problems that will interest the audience members.

TEACHING TIPS

Having described five techniques to help maintain the attention of learners in lectures, I now offer some lecture teaching tips. First, consider audiovisual aids. These aids can be helpful because people generally remember 20% of what they hear, 30% of what they see, and 50% of what they both hear and see (Howe, 1977). What aid is most often used in medical lectures? The 35mm slide! It is also the most abused. In fact, in most medical lectures I have seen over the years, slides hinder rather than help. The main reason is that the lights are turned off, which provides a setting conducive to sleep. When slides are properly prepared, the color contrast should be sufficient to allow that some lights can be kept on. If slides cannot be seen with all the lights on and if the lecture room allows only for all the lights to be fully on or fully off *slides should not be used.*

The biggest problem with slide design is the word slide that has more than 35 words. These slides are too busy to be read and may well be perturbing to the audience. Also, unless letters and numbers are at least

1/15th the height of the slide, they will not be read. The "35-word" rule and the "1/15th" rule usually are violated when speakers bring a journal article or book chapter to the medical illustration office and say, "Make me a slide of that table (or chart or graph)." In such cases, one should identify what is important on the table, chart, or graph and *simplify* it. Work with an artist in the medical illustration office to design and make a slide that shows exactly what you want the audience to see. *Several* slides may be needed to extrapolate information from one published table or illustration. Because of the frequent use of slides, I suggest that a speaker ask his medical library or medical illustration office for a copy of the guidelines published by the National Medical Audiovisual Center (1976).

Next, let's consider some other lecture-teaching tips. What about the speaker's voice? Although one should not become overly anxious about his voice, reviewing the anatomy involved in human speech production would be helpful. As we know, four phases are necessary in the production of speech: respiration, vibration, resonation, and articulation.

> Within the larynx, stretched betweent he cartilages, are the vocal folds. The compressed air from the lungs presses against the vocal folds, causing a vibration that produces sound. This sound is further resonated in the air chambers in the throat, mouth, and sinuses in the cheek bones, forehead, and nasal cavities. Finally, the sounds that have been produced and amplified are borken up by the articulators—the tongue, lips, teeth, jaw, hard and soft palates—into . . . sounds of the consonants, interspersed by the relatively free flow of air in the production of the vowel sounds. (Penner, 1984 p. 141)

A good speaking voice is produced by the proper use of all four areas: diaphragmatic breathing, a relaxed throat, an ample amount of resonation, and flexible articulators. Shallow breathing results in too low a volume an dinunplanned pauses ins peaking as air is gulped. Tense vocal cords result in an unnaturally high-pitched voice. If the resonating chambers are clogged, denasality results, and if they are overused, nasality results. Inflexible articulators will produce unclear speech sounds (Penner, 1984). Although consciously thinking of these mechanics is not advisable while one is lecturing, I do recommend that the speaker take a moment or two before lecturing to sit down, take a few relaxed breaths, and gather his thoughts. This preparation will likely make speech production more normal.

The major principle of good public speaking is to be conversational. This means emphatically that one does *not read* a presentation to the audience. Instead, the lecture is delivered as if the speaker were telling a story to one person. An outline or a few notes can be helpful. Although some presenters prefer to bring a script with them, intending to use it for reference, not for reading, I have observed that when the script is there, one tends to begin to read it.

Here are specific suggestions: Use natural hand gestures and do not remain behind a podium, walk toward the audience for emphasis, and, occasionally, speak from the side of the room. Even try walking up the side aisle. On the other hand, avoid pacing back and forth like a caged tiger. Look at the listeners, one at a time. For a moement or two, focus on one person. In doing so, look for feedback. Does that student understand what is being said? Is that person interested in the material? Does the learner appear to be actively listening and considering what it all means? This nonverbal feedback can be useful because it can help the speaker adjust the pace and content of the presentation.

The downfall for some speakers is a distracting mannerism, for example, clearing the throat or jiggling a piece of chalk. I suggest a colleague be asked to watch one lecture with the sole purpose of detecting any annoying mannerism. If such a mannerism is noted, these four steps are suggest to rid onself of it:

1. Mentally rehearse an upcoming lecture and imagine making the presentation without the undesirable behavior.
2. Create a mental image to help stop the mannerism. For example, if tugging one's hair is a habit, imagine that the hair is razor sharp and must not be touched.
3. Write on the elcture outline or notes, "I will not . . . (e.g., touch my hair)" and look at that statement during the presentation.
4. Ask a colleague to again observe a lecture and comment on whether progress has been made.

If one tries these four steps, gradual improvement should be expected, rather than extinction of the distracting mannerism in one lecture.

Mental rehearsal, even if a speaker has no unwanted behaviors, is helpful for all lecturers. As is generally known, athletes too have usually found mental rehearsal helpful. In fact, this is one of the basic principles of sports psychology. By mentally, as well as actually, practicing lectures, a speaker will increase his confidence. When one is more confident about the lecture material and about its presentation, the lecture can be altered freely, be given more spontaneously, and the unexpected responded to more adroitly.

A few comments are in order about a special type of lecture that residents help plan: grand rounds. Some physicians believe that grand rounds no longer live up to the standards of the past (Ingelfinger, 1978). Many years ago, groups of physicians walked through the wards, stopping at the bedside of each patient presenting an interesting case and commenting on the patient's care. When the trail of white coats became too large for the wards, grand rounds were moved to the hospital amphitheater, to which the patient with a timely problem was brought. Today, patients are rarely brought to grand rounds. Instead, a "case" is presented. A common criticism is that often the case is incidental to the presentation, a vestigial organ in the body of lecture.

I would prefer that grand rounds address specific patient problems. Selected cases should highlight the interconnectedness of social, economic, psychological, and physical problems, that is, the "biopsychosocial" approach advocated by Engel (1965). One should elicit audience participation, welcome their questions, and ask for their comments and criticisms. A good technique is to withhold until later the results that reveal the final diagnosis and treatment plan, meanwhile inviting audience members to problem-solve. Grand rounds will live up to the greatness of the past when it centers on problem-oriented discussion rather than on topical lectures indistinguishable from other medical school lectures.

CONCLUSION

One should become more creative in planning and presenting lectures. Creative teachers are both useful in what they teach and novel in how they teach it. Lecturers whose information is useful but not flavored with any novelty are pedantic bores. Those whose methods are novel, but whose material is not useful, are charlatans. To those who worry that I am recommending that they become entertainers, let me respond by asking for an agreement: I won't defend the charlatans if you won't defend the pedantic bores!

Our potential to become more creative teachers is highlighted by the sotry about the artist who won first prize at an art fair. When the judge gave her the award, she replied, "You know, I didn't submit my best work." The surprised judge asked her why not. She responded, "Because I haven't done it yet." None of us have done our best teaching . . . yet.

CHAPTER 6

A Review of Clinical Teaching Improvement Methods and a Theoretical Framework For Their Evaluation

KELLEY M. SKEFF
JUDITH BERMAN
GEORGETTE STRATOS

Medical educators interested in improving the quality of residents' teaching are faced with a key question: Which teaching improvement methods may be useful for these teachers? The literature already contains reviews of the effectiveness of faculty development programs in nonmedical areas (Levinson-Rose and Menges, 1981) and in the health professions in particular (Stritter, 1983). In general, these programs have been designed for teachers at the faculty level. Although the teaching settings and emphases of residents may differ from those of faculty (Tremonti and Biddle, 1982), we believe that the basic commonalities of the teaching role make existing faculty development programs relevant to teachers in general, including residents. It is our position that theoretical perspectives from education and psychology can offer important contributions toward the development of more effective methods for training teachers of clinical medicine. Therefore, the purpose of this chapter is twofold: (1) to familiarize readers with a variety of previously developed teaching improvement methods which have been used, and (2) to guide readers in a logical, theoretically based approach to the assessment and selection of methods that may be most useful in their own institutions.

METHODS OF IMPROVING TEACHING

Several formats have been used in the literature to organize discussion of the available teaching improvement methods. In reviewing teaching improvement methods for higher education, Levinson-Rose and Menges (1981) used five categories: (1) grants for faculty projects, (2) workshops and seminars, (3) feedback from student ratings, (4) microteaching practice with feedback, and (5) concept-based training with protocol materials. In his review of faculty development in the health professions, Stritter (1983) based his analysis on the scheme of Centra (1976), and included three categories: (1) technical assistance (methods involving an educational specialist), (2) high faculty involvement (methods requiring concentrated faculty time, such as workshops and seminars), and (3) structured institutional approaches (methods involving institutional sponsorship of good teaching).

Although these and other approaches provide useful categorization schemes, they do not adequately distinguish the various methods from one another. One problem is that a single teaching improvement method may incorporate several different components designed to improve teaching. For example, a seminar may include discussion with an educational consultant as well as videotape review. In addition, methods within several of the categories used by Levinson-Rose and Menges may share a specific component. For example, workshops, seminars, and interpretation of student ratings may all include consultation with a specialist in education. As a result, it is not always possible to determine the effectiveness of each specific component.

In this chapter we analyze various teaching improvement methods in terms of their different components. By considering the components separately, we believe that readers will be better able to design or select teaching improvement methods appropriate for their own institutions. The components to be covered in this chapter are (1) feedback from student ratings, (2) peer evaluation, (3) consultation with a professional educator, (4) videotape review, (5) self-evaluation, (6) concept-based training, and (7) various types of seminars and workshops that are combinations of these components. The components will be discussed in terms of their use and evaluation in both medical and other educational settings. Table 14.2 (pp. 234–235) summarizes this discussion.

Feedback from Student Ratings

Feedback from students to teachers is one of the most commonly used methods of teaching improvement. Feedback usually consists of a computerized or typewritten form filled out by learners to evaluate a teacher's performance on specified items. Informing teachers about the perceptions and judgments of their students would seem to be an appropriate method to motivate and guide teachers to improve their teaching effectiveness. However, teachers may perceive the opinions of students as threatening or they may not regard students as valid judges of teaching performance. In such situations, feedback from students may lose its potential for assisting teachers to improve.

Few studies conducted in the clinical teaching setting have examined the effects of written student feedback alone as a method of teaching improvement, and, to our knowledge, none has been directed specifically to residents' teaching. Rous et al. (1972) provided written feedback from student ratings to 27 clinical faculty, 16 of whom were then reevaluated 1 to 3 months later. The investigators reported improvement in the follow-up ratings; however, they commented that many faculty chose not to participate. Therefore, the improved ratings may not represent a general effectiveness of the method for all clinical faculty. Stillman et al. (1983) examined the effect of feedback from students, along with peer evaluation, on lecturers in a clinical pathology course. Based on improvement in student ratings from one year to the next, these authors concluded that student feedback can be an effective way of improving teaching skills. Because peer evaluation was also included in this study, the effect of student feedback alone is not clear.

As one part of an experimental study of a clinical teaching improvement methods, the results of student and house staff evaluations of their teachers were provided to attending physicians at the midpoint of a 1-month ward-attending rotation (Skeff, 1983). At the end of the rotation, ratings made by students and house staff showed no statistically significant differences between the group of attending physicians who received the midrotation ratings and a control group who did not. In addition, only 50% of the attending physicians receiving the written feedback rated it useful. Although one cannot make definitive conclusions from these few studies, the findings suggest that written student feedback alone may not be a consistently effective method for improving clinical teaching.

Evaluations of student feedback conducted in higher education settings outside of medicine indicate variability in the effectiveness of written student feedback to improve teaching (Rotem and Glasman, 1979). Several approaches have been developed to enhance the effectiveness of student feedback. Pambookian (1976) and Centra (1973) combined student ratings with teacher self-assessments so that teachers could compare their own views of their teaching with those of their students. They found that, over time, teachers tended to receive improved ratings on those items for which there had been initial discordance between the teacher's self-ratings and the student ratings. That is, when a teacher's self-ratings on an item were higher than those ratings made by students on that item, the teacher was more likely to improve that aspect of teaching.

Research by Aleamoni (1978) and McKeachie (1979) found that having an educational consultant review students' feedback with instructors also appeared to enhance the usefulness of this method. The consultant may be able to provide teachers with interpretations of the student ratings that increase their apparent validity and also guide the teachers in using the ratings to improve teaching. To avoid the need for an educational consultant, Cohen and Herr (1982) developed a method in which faculty received student ratings along with a programmed feedback booklet designed to help them review, interpret, and utilize the student ratings. Although students' end-of-term ratings did not indicate that this method was significantly more effective than other student feedback approaches, the teachers' self-ratings appeared to favor this method, possibly because it may improve teachers' confidence in their teaching abilities.

In summary, student feedback by itself does not appear to be a consistently effective method to improve teaching. However, the additional use of educational consultants, self-assessments, or booklets to guide a teacher's interpretation and use of student ratings may improve the effectiveness of this method. Because of its relative ease of implementation and its increased effectiveness when combined with other components, student feedback as a teaching improvement method for residents deserves further study.

Peer Review

Peer observation and review by faculty as methods for teaching improvement have adequate precedent in medical training. Having colleagues and faculty observe and review one's clinical work is a common practice in clinical instruction. In addition, the observation of peers is a method of learning often used by house staff and students.

Although most studies of peer review of teaching in higher education focus on peer evaluation for administrative purposes, findings from these studies have important implications even for those considering the implementation of peer review as a method for teaching improvement. The first major finding of these studies is that colleagues may be generous in their ratings of peers, thereby limiting the potential validity and helpfulness of the evaluation. Second, the interrater reliability of peer ratings made by different colleagues can be relatively low. Although poor interrater reliability should not preclude the use of peer ratings for teaching improvement, studies of reliability make it clear that different observers may give quite different ratings of the same teacher. Centra (1975) concluded that colleague ratings of classroom teaching behavior generally do not have adequate reliability for tenure and promotion decisions. He noted, however, that both training the peer observers and increasing the number of observations might increase the reliability of the ratings. A third important finding regarding peer review is that getting peers to review their colleagues' teaching can be difficult. This may not be as large a problem for residents as for university faculty, but with their busy schedules residents may also resist conducting peer review.

The literature on the use of peer review for teaching improvement in higher education reveals some positive findings. Sweeney and Grasha (1978) reported on a program in which volunteer trios of faculty collaborated to discuss educational issues and to arrange to observe each others' classes. The members of the team were trained by a teaching development specialist. After observing others, these faculty then met to discuss their observations as a trio, emphasizing teaching strengths as well as problems. Faculty reported gaining insights both from being observed and observing. In addition, faculty reported they were able to consider and implement the suggestions of colleagues in this program. In his review of peer evaluation, Sell (1986) noted the positive potential of peer review; however, he also pointed out a lack of consistent evidence of the effectiveness of peer review as a method to improve teacher performance. In summary, the literature in higher education indicates that peer review may be a useful method for improving teaching, although those using this method should be aware of the significant problems associated with it.

Having peers critique teaching performance has been infrequently studied in clinical teaching. One study conducted in the clinical setting abilities of observation, greater awareness of student needs, and more conscious acceptance of teaching strengths and weaknesses. However, this study also indicated potential sources of resistance to peer review. In this study, peer review was perceived by some teachers as judgmental or biased, thus showing the potentially threatening nature of peer review to these teachers. These authors also pointed out the difficulty in identifying faculty to observe others.

As part of a study of a teaching improvement method for attending physicians, Skeff (1981) asked participating attending physicians whether they would be willing to have colleagues review videotapes of their own teaching performance with them. Nearly 100% of the participants in that study stated a willingness to have another attending physician act as a facilitator for reviewing their videotape, thus indicating a willingness to have peer review at some level. Over 80% of participants also stated a willingness to have the head of their department facilitate a review of videotapes of their teaching. The apparent acceptance of peer review by these clinical teachers may have been due to the specific non-threatening approach used in this study. It is also possible that the positive attitudes of these attending physicians may not be a valid indicator of whether they would actually participate in this or other peer review methods. Their responses, however, suggest acceptance of peer review by attending physicians.

Although there has been relatively little formal study of the use of peer review methods for improving the teaching of residents, some research indicates the positive potential for this method. Medio et al. (Chapter 13 in this volume; Table 13.1, p. 220) used peer review in three of four teaching sessions. The participants evaluated the peer feedback as one of the most useful aspects of the instruction. With small groups of second-year residents, Edwards et al. (Chapter 9, p. 173) reviewed teaching videotapes. The residents who received this peer review were evaluated significantly higher on teaching skills by trained raters than residents who were not critiqued.

Residents in training may already recognize the important roles they play in teaching and learning from peers; therefore, assuming a role in the improvement of each others' teaching may not require a major change in mind set. On the other hand, residents may have difficulty reviewing and commenting on the teaching of their peers or accepting their peers' comments on their own teaching. Further study would be important to assess resident attitudes toward peer review. In addition, although not truly peer review, the use of faculty as "peer" reviewers of residents' teaching deserves consideration. Because residents may residents' teaching deserves consideration. Since residents may already expect to receive comments from faculty on their medical knowledge and abilities, they may also be willing to accept faculty comments on their teaching. The effectiveness of faculty review as an approach to teaching improvement for residents needs to be studied.

In sum, although the literature does not allow one to predict the effectiveness of peer review for improving teaching, some studies suggest its usefulness to residents. If peer review is used, training the residents as observers and critics of teaching, as well as making certain that the review criteria are agreed upon in advance, may enhance the usefulness of this teaching improvement approach.

Consultation with a Professional Educator

In education, as in other fields, a professional consultant can provide special expertise. Such expertise can be provided through observation of a teacher followed by a private consultation, a group meeting, a videotape review, or other methods. With regard to clinical teaching, professional educators may be able to provide (a) knowledge of important educational theories that bear on clinical teaching, (b) expertise in teaching skills, (c) expertise related to different approaches to teaching, such as computer-aided instruction, (d) knowledge of techniques to assist a teacher in analyzing his own teaching.

In Stritter's review of faculty development programs in medicine (1983), several methods of educational consultation are discussed. Studies by Foley et al. (1976) and Irby et al. (1976) represent two different uses of consultation with educators to improve faculty lecturing. The first study included videotaping lectures of faculty, having faculty assess their own lecturing abilities, and having them rate their own videotape using specified criteria. Educational consultants also rated the videotapes and then provided written feedback to the teachers. In addition, the educators conducted group sessions for all the participating teachers. It is important to note that two of the major activities of the consultant in this approach, that is, reviewing the videotape and providing written consultation, did not require one-on-one contact with the consultant; thus, aspects of this method could provide an easily implementable, self-contained approach, which avoids the time limitations of individual teacher-consultant meetings. In contrast, Irby and his associates (1976) conducted consultant observations of faculty lectures and provided immediate verbal and written feedback to the faculty. In a similar manner, Patridge, Harris, and Petzel (1980) observed tutors in an introduction to clinical medicine course, and provided feedback regarding their clinical teaching. These approaches appeared to have positive effects on teacher performance.

In addition to working with individuals, consultants may be used to conduct faculty development efforts with groups, such as workshops, retreats, seminars, and the like. Wergin, Mason, and Munson (1976) reported on their experience as educational consultants in a medical center. They pointed out potential pitfalls in consultation, such as the lack of adequate knowledge by the consultant of faculty expectations or needs, and the lack of adequate credibility and trust of the consultant. Based on their successful and unsuccessful experiences, they provided guidelines that may increase the likelihood of successful use of a consultant, including their belief that a consultant should move from a professional-expert phase to a personal collaborative phase. In summary, the literature indicates that the use of educational consultants can be an effective approach to improving clinical teaching.

Videotape Review

Videotape is recognized as a powerful tool for the observation, discussion, and improvement of teaching. In general, videotape can be used by teachers in two major ways: (1) to review their own performance either with or without others, and (2) to review previously collected or developed tapes as stimuli for discussion of effective and ineffective teaching approaches. As a method of teaching improvement, videotape review has been shown to have potential to affect teachers' attitudes, knowledge, and skills.

The viewing of videotapes can influence attitudes in at least two major ways. First, in the self-confrontation promoted by reviewing videotapes of one's own behavior, perceived discrepancies between the observed performance and the internal standards of the viewer can create dissatisfaction that motivates a desire to change behavior. This phenomenon is consistent with dissonance theory (Festinger, 1957), which postulates that the discovery of discrepancies between observed behavior and intentions or goals is a motivating force to reduce the discrepancies by changing self-perception, behavior, or both (see Chapter 4, pp. 63–65). In addition, a videotape review of one's own or another's behavior may make a person more confident in his ability to perform a given behavior, and thereby increase his drive to perform that behavior. This phenomenon is consistent with self-efficacy theory (Bandura, 1977), which relates the belief that one can perform some defined behavior (i.e., one's self-efficacy) to the likelihood that the behavior will be accomplished. Thus, by either making a teacher less content with his teaching behavior or making a teacher feel more confident about his ability to perform effective teaching behaviors, videotape review can affect teacher attitudes. (It should be noted that videotape review might also lead to a decreased level of confidence in teaching ability, thereby diminishing drive to perform a given behavior.)

Videotape review can also affect teacher knowledge, for example by (1) increasing teachers' understanding of themselves and others or (2) increasing teachers' knowledge of educational concepts. In the method of Interpersonal Process Recall developed by Kagan (1975), two or more participants who have been videotaped (e.g., a teacher and one or more students) review the tape with a trained facilitator. With the guidance of the facilitator, the participants recall and discuss the thoughts and feelings that occurred during the videotaped interaction, thereby gaining insight into their behavior and gaining knowledge about themselves. In addition to learning about themselves, teachers can review videotaped examples of teaching skills as a mechanism to increase their knowledge of educational concepts underlying the teaching process. Gliessman and Pugh (1978a, 1978b) have shown that viewing filmed examples of teaching behaviors as part of a method to teach educational concepts can increase the knowledge of those educational concepts related to the behaviors. This deeper understanding of the conceptual basis for teaching skills can be advantageous to the teacher in choosing appropriate teaching approaches.

In addition to influencing attitudes and knowledge, videotape review can have a positive impact on skill acquisition. In fact, because of the extensive, and successful, implementation of microteaching, skill acquisition may represent the most common use of videotape in teacher training. Microteaching is a method for the practice and critique of directly observable teaching skills (Allen and Ryan, 1969). Participants in this method practice teaching short lessons with students or peers. The practice lesson is taped and played back immediately so that the presenter and other participants can discuss the skills practiced during the episode.

Although videotape review is a powerful technique for reviewing one's own or others' behavior, there are several potential negative effects and difficulties associated with its use. First, videotape review may be threatening to participants. Simply viewing oneself on videotape can be a stressful experience. As a result, some teachers may not wish to participate. Second, emotional response to videotape review may inhibit the acquisition of knowledge or skills. Third, if videotape review leads the viewers to perceive their performance as deficient, they may have lowered confidence in their ability to teach. This negative effect may not only decrease teachers' motivation to change their teaching, but may even decrease the desire to teach at all.

Relevant to the potential drawbacks of videotape review, Perlberg (1983, p 647), focusing on video self-confrontation, emphasizes that successful videotape review depends on the effectiveness of the consultant who facilitates the review, and the quality and degree of his intervention. He states that "One cannot emphasize too strongly the importance of acquiring the necessary consultancy skills for effective use of video self-confrontation in higher education" (p 658).

In their extensive review of videotape playback in teacher education, Fuller and Manning (1973) make recommendations for increasing the likelihood of successful use of this method, including (a) select a "typical" performance for review, (b) ensure a psychologically safe playback environment, (c) facilitate a teacher's identification of deficiencies, and (d) provide feedback on the videotaped performance that is unambiguous and related to clear performance goals set before the videotape review. Although these guidelines can facilitate the success of this method, we believe that those who choose to use this method should: (1) recognize its potential for creating powerful positive and negative effects in the participants and (2) consider the need for acquiring expertise for implementing the method appropriately.

Videotape review has been used in numerous studies of methods to improve clinical teaching (e.g., Bazuin and Yonke, 1978; Cassie et al., 1977; Foley et al., 1976; Mahler and Benor, 1984; Sheets and Henry, 1984; Skeff, 1983; Skeff et al., 1986). In addition, several studies to improve residents' teaching have also incorporated videotape review (Chapter 9 of this volume; Jewett et al., 1982b; Lawson and Harvill, 1980; Meleca and Schimpfhauser, 1976). Most of these investigators used videotape review as only one of several components in more complex methods such as seminars or workshops, combining it with consultation, self-assessment, group discussions, microteaching, and other techniques. In general, the evaluations of such methods with residents showed positive effects on resident's teaching skills, indicating the usefulness of this method for the improvement of clinical teaching by both attending physicians and residents.

Self-Evaluation

Self-evaluation has great intuitive appeal as a method to improve teaching. As noted by Seldin (1980, p. 85), an opportunity for self-reflection, without fear of retribution no matter what is revealed, can lead to the resolution of problems and the implementation of methods to improve teaching skills. It could be argued that professionals should undertake periodic self-evaluation for the purpose of ongoing improvement. However, clinical teachers, including residents and faculty, seldom use self-evaluation in any formal way as a method of improving their teaching.

Self-evaluation can take place using several methods, including self-rating forms, a review of videotapes or audiotapes of one's teaching interaction, or observation of colleagues for the purpose of comparison with one's teaching (Carroll, 1981). Although the term self-evaluation implies an independent activity of the teacher, self-analysis by itself appears to have only limited promise for improving teaching (Seldin, 1980, p.85). Teachers may not know how to evaluate their performance or they may not know how to respond to problems revealed by the evaluation. Therefore, several approaches have been developed to increase the usefulness of self-evaluation to teachers.

First, a commonly discussed method for using self-evaluation is to have the teacher complete a self-rating on the same form being used by his students. This self-assessment provides the opportunity for the teacher to then compare his self-ratings with the ratings of students. As mentioned in the section on student ratings, empirical findings indicate that instructors will focus on and improve their performance on those items on which the teacher's self-ratings are higher than the students' ratings (Pambookian, 1976). Apparently, teachers are motivated to address the specific behaviors pinpointed by the discrepancies between their own and their students' ratings.

Second, the use of a facilitator to guide a teacher's review of videotapes of his own teaching performance provides another powerful means of enhancing self-evaluation. A significant problem with videotape review is that it often leaves instructors wondering exactly what it is that they are supposed to look for on the videotape (Carroll, 1981). Using a facilitator to guide the review by focusing on specific incidents or behaviors can improve the effectiveness of this technique for self-evaluation and teaching improvement (Seldin, 1980, p. 86).

Few, if any, studies of clinical teaching have used self-evaluation as the sole method for teaching improvement. Although comparisons of teacher self- ratings with ratings of students, review of videotapes with a facilitator (Skeff, 1983; Skeff et al., 1986) and self-review of videotapes (Foley et al., 1976; Lawson and Harvill, 1980) have been studied, they have been used in combination with other approaches to teaching improvement. Therefore, although one would assume that self-evaluation could play a valuable role, its specific contribution to the improvement of clinical teaching is not known.

Concept-Based Training

Concept-based training refers to programs aimed at improving teachers' understanding of the concepts underlying teaching skills: concepts about the nature, purposes, and limits of various teaching approaches (Gliessman and Pugh, 1984). Underlying concept-based teacher training programs is the assumption that more in-depth knowledge about the conceptual basis for teaching behaviors can lead not only to increases in teacher knowledge but also to changes in teacher performance.

Gliessman and Pugh (1978a) showed that concept acquisition was more effective when teacher trainees not only studied definitions of concepts, but also viewed films showing examples of teaching behaviors representing the concepts. In another study, these authors showed that higher concept scores were achieved when trainees had the opportunity to discuss the filmed instances of the concepts than without such discussion (Gliessman and Pugh, 1978b). Recently, these authors have shown that teachers can change performance of specific behaviors when the concept-based training includes only discussions to clarify teachers' conceptualizations of teaching behaviors, without the use of filmed examples from the training (Gliessman and Pugh, 1984).

Skeff et al. (1986) studied a concept-based seminar method to teach about educational concepts relevant to clinical teaching. This method included a facilitated discussion of videotaped reenactments of clinical teaching episodes in order to familiarize attending physicians with educational concepts such as evaluation, feedback. Analysis of questionnaire data and ratings of videotapes of actual teaching performance revealed that the method improved attending physicians' attitudes and teaching performance. To date, there have been no studies of the effectiveness of concept-based training as a method to improve teaching by residents; however, given the success of this approach with attending physicians, it is likely that such programs could have positive results for residents as well.

Another type of concept-based instruction that has not been adequately studied is the use of written material about teaching concepts and behaviors, both with and without discussion. Because of the abundance of literature on clinical teaching as well as teaching handbooks for residents (Schwenk and Whitman, 1984), formal studies of this approach to improving residents' teaching are needed.

Multicomponent Methods: Seminars and Workshops

As mentioned previously in this chapter, few of the components described above have been studied in clinical teaching as methods in and of themselves. In general, teaching improvement methods used for residents and clinical faculty have represented various combinations of the above-described approaches. In this section, we describe a few of these multicomponent methods that have been found to have a positive impact on teacher performance.

Mahler and Benor (1984) reported the positive effects of a 4-day teacher-training workshop on clinical faculty teaching behavior. This study was unique in that it measured long-term impacts on teaching activity and found that effects of the workshop lasted for up to six months before showing decline. This workshop emphasized the type of videotape review used in microteaching, but it also included peer-feedback, self-evaluation of videotapes, and private consultation/discussions with a tutor-consultant. Skeff et al. (1986) conducted two-hour seminars that combined the facilitated review of videotape re- enactments of actual episodes of clinical teaching as a method of concept-based training, along with feedback from student ratings and faculty self-assessment using the same rating form used by students. This approach resulted in positive impacts on the attitudes and teaching behaviors of attending physicians on inpatient wards.

Several multicomponent programs have been conducted to improve resident teaching. Lawson and Harvill (1980) conducted a program of three 1-hour sessions that included lecture-discussion activity, videotape review with microteaching, peer feedback, use of a consultant, and self-evaluations. This program resulted in measurable positive changes in attitude and teaching skills. Jewett et al. (1982b) studied a program of 9 hours of workshops for residents including videotape review of approaches typically taken to teaching, individual and group review of videotapes of participants' teaching, and group and individual feedback sessions regarding evaluations of the residents' teaching by faculty, peers, and students. This approach resulted in reports from participants of increased confidence in teaching, increased levels of positive feedback on participants' teaching, and increased ratings of teaching effectiveness by faculty, students, and peers. In Chapter 9, Edwards et al. describe conducting a half-day workshop during the first year of residency and peer review sessions of videotapes during the second year. Evaluations of the videotapes by trained raters showed significant improvement for experimental residents compared with a matched control group.

Three additional programs are described in the case studies of this volume. Camp and Hoban (Chapter 12) conducted four 2-hour instructional sessions about lecturing, informal teaching, psychomotor skills, and case presentations using a variety of methods in each session.

Meleca and Pearsol (Chapter 11) taught a 1-day workshop to surgery residents. Medio et al. (Chapter 13) taught four sessions dealing with lecturing, giving feedback, questioning techniques, and teaching on work rounds. The evaluation of these programs, which mainly consisted of asking for participant's opinions, indicated that the methods generally appeared to have positive results.

In this section we have reviewed several approaches for improving teaching. As discussed, these approaches incorporate a variety of dimensions. For example, some approaches involve providing teachers with feedback regarding their performance, and others offer a conceptually based orientation to teaching improvement, whereas yet others take a practical skills approach to training. It appears that many of the single-component methods, such as student evaluation and peer evaluation, have not been shown to be consistently effective. The most convincing evidence for effectiveness comes from the studies of multicomponent approaches. However, when combined, the relative contribution of each component is not known. Therefore, we do not wish to imply that one of these approaches is necessarily superior to the others or should be considered more widely applicable across all educational circumstances. The lack of empirical studies comparing individual components and comparing combinations of the components in medical and nonmedical settings does not allow specific recommendations as to the most appropriate method for residents. In addition, the selection of a teaching improvement method may frequently be dependent on practical constraints such as the degree of institutional support, availability of educational experts, and availability of residents' time. Thus, the most appropriate method may vary across institutions because of different needs and different resources.

In the absence of clear guidelines from empirical studies, those involved in the design and selection of teaching improvement methods for residents might be assisted by guidelines based on theoretical grounds. However, there has been little attention paid to providing a theoretical basis for comparison of these methods. The field of faculty development lacks a single, cohesive and widely accepted theoretical framework for conceptualizing and evaluating methods for the improvement of teaching. However, a variety of theoretical perspectives do exist that can offer insights into the process of teaching improvement. These perspectives may be useful to those individuals selecting from available teaching improvement approaches as well as those developing new methods for meeting residents' teaching improvement needs. We turn to a discussion of these theoretical perspectives in the next section.

THEORETICALLY BASED GUIDELINES FOR EVALUATING METHODS TO IMPROVE RESIDENTS' TEACHING

In this section, we discuss a variety of theories relevant to teaching improvement methods. In addition, we present a set of theoretically based questions to guide educators in making creative choices among methods or designing new approaches. We have drawn upon different, and in some cases competing, educational and psychological theories that we believe to be relevant to important issues regarding teaching improvement methods.

A set of theory-based questions are provided as guides for the reader's consideration. It should not be assumed that a teaching improvement method that does not embody a particular theoretical principle is necessarily ineffective. Rather, we believe that the incorporation of these theoretical principles can enhance the likelihood of residents' learning during a teaching improvement method. Subscription to one or another theoretical perspective may lead different readers to follow a different particular set of guidelines in designing a teaching improvement program for residents.

We have organized these questions around three fundamental and interrelated areas of learning: the acquisition of attitudes, knowledge, and skills (Bloom, 1956a, b). Some teaching improvement methods may focus on improving attitudes toward the teaching process; others may enhance teachers' knowledge of educational principles or the content area they expect to teach; whereas other methods may concentrate on providing teachers with specific teaching skills. Methods to improve teaching may focus on any or all of these dimensions.

For the purpose of this chapter, we have limited the number of theoretically based questions that might be asked about a teaching improvement method. Because it would be unrealistic to cover all theoretical perspectives, we have selected and summarized the essence of key perspectives that we believe provide a foundation for developing guidelines for teaching improvement methods. Our intent is not to provide an exhaustive, or even comprehensive, compilation of theoretical questions, but rather to begin to establish a theoretical basis to guide the future design, selection, and evaluation of methods of teaching improvement.

We have tried to keep in mind a broad range of needs so that these questions will be applicable across a variety of situations. For example, the educator who only seeks to use a brief intervention for improving the teaching of residents should find ideas to guide the selection of a brief method. At the other end of the spectrum, the program director with a mandate to establish, or revise, a full-scale teaching improvement program may wish to make a more extensive application of the guidelines. The remainder of this chapter includes two major sections. In the first we discuss theories pertaining to attitudes. In the second, we discuss theories related to the acquisition of knowledge and skills.

ATTITUDES

Teacher attitudes are critical to the success of teaching improvement methods at several levels including: teachers' initial motivation to participate in the method, their desire to improve teaching performance, and their attitudes regarding, and dedication to, the teaching role. It is important to examine whether teaching improvement methods take into account relevant educational and psychological theory in fostering positive teacher attitudes. Although the discussion of attitudes could be approached from several perspectives, in this chapter we are primarily focusing on issues of teacher motivation, including theories of need, motive acquisition, self-efficacy, and adult learning that have relevance to the process of selecting teaching improvement methods.

QUESTION 1: Does the teaching improvement method address the residents' perceived needs, including their interest in teaching improvement?

Need Theory

In the selection of a teaching improvement method, assessing the needs and initial attitudes of the prospective participants can be critical. The degree to which a method for improving residents' teaching captures the interest, trust, acceptance and enthusiasm of these residents is likely to influence the eventual success or failure of that method.

According to Maslow's (1954) hierarchy of needs, individuals must satisfy lower-order needs (e.g., sleep or food) before they will be motivated toward higher-level achievements (e.g., personal growth). Additionally, psychological stress is likely to result when individuals are placed in situations that do not allow them to gratify their needs. Since most residents might view teaching improvement as a means to personal growth, rather than satisfaction of basic needs, it is likely to be considered a higher-order need. Because teacher training does not form an established part of the medical education system, residents do not generally expect to undergo a systematic course of study to acquire

Since most residents might view teaching improvement as a means to personal growth, rather than satisfaction of basic needs, it is likely to be considered a higher-order need. Because teacher training does not form an established part of the medical education system, residents do not generally expect to undergo a systematic course of study to acquire proficiency as teachers of medicine. In addition, residents have multiple and demanding responsibilities, leaving them with little time to think about or improve their teaching. The pressures inherent in a resident's role may be more likely to promote resistant attitudes toward participation in teaching improvement methods rather than to encourage an interest in the improvement of teaching. The literature on faculty development in higher education outside of medicine provides extensive documentation of faculty resistance to teaching improvement methods (Gaff, 1976). This resistance may occur because faculty who want to survive in the academic environment may be forced to satisfy more immediate needs before they can attend to their growth as teachers. Thus, need theory indicates the importance of knowing a teacher's attitudes toward the improvement of teaching, that is, whether they view it as the pursuance of primary or secondary needs. Although research has not clearly documented the attitudes of residents toward the process of teaching improvement, resistance is possible among this group of teachers.

In summary, need theory implies that educators who are responsible for designing or selecting a method for improving the teaching done by residents should evaluate residents' attitudes toward teaching improvement. This evaluation can be either formal or informal, and should focus on determining the degree of interest and willingness among residents to focus on issues of teaching. Such a survey can strengthen the design of the teaching program by ensuring that it meets the perceived needs of the residents involved and by identifying and addressing resistant attitudes in advance of implementing the program. Before using a method such as student feedback, peer evaluation, self-evaluation, or even one of the more complex multicomponent methods, knowledge of residents' perceived needs as teachers can allow one to address such needs. In addition, if residents are resistant to participation, attempting to use methods that are clearly relevant to their actual teaching may decrease resistance.

QUESTION 2: Does the method assist residents in conceptualizing their teaching role and in assessing their priorities as teachers?

Motive Acquisition Theory

If evaluation of residents' attitudes indicates suboptimal motivation toward teaching improvement, an effective teaching improvement method needs to incorporate approaches to increase residents' motivation to improve teaching. While need theory focuses on identifying levels of need as the sources of motivation, the theory of motive acquisition concentrates on changing an individual's belief structure. McClelland (1965) described motives as a complex hierarchy of associated beliefs that are prioritized by the individual. Recognizing that psychologists generally consider motivation a relatively stable and difficult property to change, McClelland developed and tested a program for motivational change. McClelland hypothesized that motives could be altered by a process that involved exposing an individual's beliefs and concepts underlying each motive, consciously labeling aspects of each motive, tying the motives to as many cues as possible in everyday life, and increasing the salience of some motives over others. McClelland defined several steps to accomplish attitudinal change, including self-study, goal-setting and application, and group support.

Several principles from the theory of motive acquisition hold implications for the selection of methods to train residents as teachers. First, self-study that exposes an individual's underlying beliefs and concepts can lead to motivational change. The theory of motive acquisition implies that an initial step in developing teacher motivation should focus on the teacher's conceptualization of his teaching role. Residents, like many other teachers, may be more focused on the content they teach than on their role as teachers or on the process of teaching. According to motive acquisition theory, self- analysis that results in a clear conception of the residents' teaching role can increase their motivation to improve teaching.

Any of the previously discussed teaching improvement approaches has the potential to stimulate self-analysis. However, it is possible that methods that focus on specific skills or content may not result in a consideration by residents of their personal priorities as teachers. Thus, a method may require a planned opportunity for participants to discuss their perceptions of the general meaning of teaching and its personal relevance to their careers.

QUESTION 3: Does the teaching improvement method provide residents with opportunities for setting their own teaching goals?

QUESTION 4: Does the method facilitate application of teaching goals established by the resident?

According to a second principle of the theory of motive acquisition, involving individuals in goal-setting related to a motive, followed by concrete application of the individual's goals, helps to maintain the salience of that motive. Increasing the salience of certain motives is essential for an individual to acquire those motives. Because of their multiple and competing responsibilities, residents may not have a motive to improve their teaching. Therefore, having residents define their own teaching goals ensures the salience of those goals for each resident. According to motive acquisition theory, raising teaching goals to a conscious level can motivate residents' to desire to improve their teaching. All teaching improvement methods have the potential to increase the salience of teaching in the minds of the residents. However, not all methods have the participants define their own goals as a part of the process. This theoretical principle implies the usefulness of that procedure.

In addition to setting goals, residents need evidence that changes they have applied in their teaching to achieve their goals will actually be useful. If residents can readily see the positive results of their changes, they will be more likely to dedicate themselves to an ongoing process of growth as teachers. For teachers to see the positive results of their teaching changes, a teaching improvement method should be implemented when the skills acquired can be readily applied. Thus, timing a method to occur when residents will be faced with teaching responsibilities (e.g., before a ward rotation with interns or students) can allow residents to see the results of their teaching improvement efforts. This principle is commonly overlooked. For example, a teaching improvement method such as student feedback is often given at the end of a rotation when a teacher cannot easily implement changes and see their positive results.

QUESTION 5: Does the method provide a conducive atmosphere?

Another principle drawn from McClelland's theory concerns the importance of a conducive environment to facilitating the examination and alteration of one's motives. McClelland suggests that an empathetic interpersonal climate can minimize anxiety that may be aroused by changing attitudes closely associated with an individual's self-concept. In addition, a warm atmosphere may supply positive reinforcement for personal change, and the mutual support provided by a group of individuals engaged in a similar growth process may serve to reinforce attitudinal change. Therefore, the atmosphere created in a teaching improvement method for residents takes on special importance. Almost all teaching improvement methods have the potential to be threatening rather than supportive experiences. Student evaluation, peer review, consultation with an educator, and even self-evaluation can take on a tone of criticism rather than support. Examining the atmosphere of a method may give clues to its effectiveness for attitudinal change.

QUESTION 6: Does the method foster participants' internal motivation for teaching?

Theorists concerned with motive acquisition have stressed the role of education in enhancing, rather than stifling, intrinsic motivation, that is, motivation coming from within the individual (Bates, 1979). Recognizing that, by its nature, intrinsic motivation cannot be made compulsory, Cohen (1983) suggested personal causation theory (deCharms, 1976) as a model for the development of motivation among teachers. Personal causation theory distinguishes between individuals who believe they can initiate change in their environment and individuals who believe their behavior is determined by forces beyond their control. Individuals operating under the former attitudinal framework have been characterized as (1) internally motivated, (2) able to set and carry through realistic goals, (3) taking responsibility for their own successes and failures, and (4) high in self-confidence. With regard to the selection of teaching improvement methods for residents, this theoretical perspective suggests that effective methods need to build on and reinforce residents' internal motivations for teaching.

If residents do not assume a self-motivated approach toward improving their teaching, it would appear unlikely that they would continue the process of self-evaluation and improvement with their own teaching. Research has demonstrated possible inhibiting effects of extrinsic rewards on intrinsic motivation (Deci and Ryan, 1982), suggesting that teaching awards and other methods of teaching improvement that rely strongly on external reinforcement may not foster improvement over the long run. According to this theoretical concept, a teaching improvement method should emphasize the personal (intrinsic) reasons why a resident should implement a change in his teaching. Methods should not simply emphasize the ideas of others. Although extrinsic methods such as student feedback, peer evaluation, or a consultant's advice can be used to guide a resident, the final impetus and decisions regarding change should be the responsibility of the resident.

QUESTION 7: Does the method enhance residents' perceptions of their own potential effectiveness as teachers?

Self-Efficacy Theory

Thus far, we have focused on the use of motivation to gain residents' interest and involvement in teaching improvement strategies. We now turn to the issue of assisting residents to recognize their power and potential as teachers. Self-efficacy theory, an outgrowth of motivation theory, has been used in the context of teacher training to refer to the extent to which teachers believe they have the capacity to affect student performance (Ashton, 1984). Research has shown a positive relationship between teachers' sense of efficacy and the achievement of their students.

Residents may not recognize their already present abilities as teachers, nor the importance of their teaching to students and interns. By focusing on the positive ratings on rating forms, showing models that exemplify the importance of residents as teachers, or using videotapes or role-playing to document previous or newly acquired skills, a method may increase residents' sense of self-efficacy in their skills and in their potential as teachers.

QUESTION 8: Does the method foster self-directed learning by drawing on participants' personal experience, demonstrating relevance to their needs, and using a problem-centered approach as a motivation for learning?

Adult Learning Theory

Knowles (1978) introduced the concept of andragogy, a developmental theory of adult learning based on the assumption that the factors that motivate adults to learn differ from those that motivate children. This theory, which offers principles to guide the facilitation of learning among adults, holds implications for the selection of methods to improve the teaching of residents. According to Knowles, andragogy is based on four assumptions about adult learning: (1) adults require self-direction in order to maintain a positive self-concept; (2) adults rely on their experience as an important motivation for learning; (3) adults require a defined need and a sense of relevance to learn; and (4) adults are motivated by a problem-centered, as opposed to subject- centered, approach to learning. Residents, as adult learners, can be expected to respond to teaching improvement methods that are clearly relevant to their teaching experience. As adult learners they will probably respond most readily if the method includes active learning that allows them to respond to their own problems and to set their own teaching improvement goals.

This theory would emphasize that teaching improvment methods for residents be relevant to their needs, utilize residents' experience in the process, and focus on a problem-centered approach to teaching improvement. These issues may seem most applicable to concept-based methods, seminars, or workshops. However, even for methods such as student feedback or peer evaluation, having residents involved in the development of the evaluation form can provide the opportunity to incorporate the principles of adult learning.

KNOWLEDGE AND SKILLS

In addition to influencing residents' attitudes, a teaching improvement method can focus on the acquisition of knowledge or skills. In the following section, we draw upon basic principles derived from several theories of learning, including behaviorism, social learning theory, Gestalt theory, and cognitive theory to guide educators in the design and selection of effective teaching improvement methods. There are major conceptual differences among these theories of learning. Behaviorist theories propose that learning occurs through contiguous association of events or ideas. In contrast, theories of Gestalt psychology and cognitive psychology argue that sensory data are organized according to innate perceptual processes of the mind (i.e., it is perceptually interpreted sensory data, not raw stimuli, that are learned). Finally, social learning theory can be viewed as a hybrid form of cognitive behaviorism that tries to provide a synthesis of cognitive psychology with the principles of behavioral modification.

Many learning theories are relevant to the acquisition of both knowledge and skills. Therefore, we are discussing theories related to both knowledge and skill acquisition in this section. Knowledge acquired in teaching improvement methods might include the knowledge related to the field of education (i.e., knowledge regarding the teaching process) as well as to the field of medicine (e.g., content related to disease processes). Similarly, skills instruction in a teaching improvement method might include instruction in teaching skills as well as in technical skill used in the practice of medicine.

QUESTION 9: Does the teaching improvement method include clear behavioral statements of goals for learners?

Behaviorist Theory

Behaviorism as a theory has two general forms, stimulus-response (S-R) theory (often referred to as traditional learning theory) and Skinnerian theory. S-R theory takes the position that the behavior of man can be investigated without appeals to consciousness or introspection (Watson, 1924). Thus, mental activity can only be studied as observable behaviors. S-R theory refers to the building of simple behavioral units into more complex learning structures. According to S-R theory, knowledge is composed hierarchically of little bits of knowledge. Like S-R theory, Skinnerian theory rejects explanations of behavior that appeal to inner psychic forces of any kind. Skinnerian theory refers to the shaping or control of behavior as an end in itself (Skinner, 1938).

According to theories of behaviorism, when the goals of an educational program are presented in concrete behavioral (and measurable) terms, the teacher has greater ability both to design a program that will shape the learner's behavior toward goals and to evaluate the program. Proponents of the use of behavioral objectives for educational goals emphasize the necessity of translating goals into measurable behaviors (Mager, 1972). "The translation process itself has a beneficial effect on the teacher and student alike, forcing the teacher to reflect on precisely what he or she believes is most important for the student to know, and what student behaviors will comprise evidence for his knowing those things" (Bower and Hilgard, 1981, p. 538). The issue of behavioral objectives is clearly relevant to teaching improvement methods for residents. If a method does not guide a resident to the actual teaching behaviors that can improve his teaching, the method may fall short of the goal of influencing teaching. This concern is relevant to all methods, from student feedback to the multicomponent combination methods.

QUESTION 10: Does the method provide the resident with opportunities for active learning?

Behaviorists believe that when learners actively manipulate the learning material, i.e., respond to it, write it down, and relate one part to another, they are likely to learn better (Bobrow and Bower, 1969; Slamecka and Graf, 1978). "Adults better remember information that they have had to connect actively in some prescribed way" (Bower and Hilgard, 1981, p. 539). For example, "people are most likely to learn from text if they ask questions about it, then search the text for answers, then actively recite the answers to themselves" (Bower and Hilgard, 1981, p.539).

Like other learning, mastery of information taught in a teaching improvement method can be enhanced by the active involvement of the residents, including the analysis, synthesis, and application of the educational material being taught. This principle may seem best suited for application to methods that purport to teach specific knowledge or skills, for example, concept-based methods and microteaching. However, other methods such as student feedback or peer evaluation may incorporate active interpretation and classification of the results of the ratings. Thus, asking whether a method incorporates active learning is probably appropriate for any teaching improvement method.

QUESTION 11: Is the material being taught in the teaching-improvement method organized according to levels of complexity?

The hierarchical task analysis proposed by Gagné (1978) argues that complex educational tasks or skills can be broken down into a hierarchy of elementary behavioral components or subskills. According to Gagné, the hierarchy suggests the progression in which subskills should be taught. For example, presentation of a learning situation for each new skill should be preceded by mastery of subordinate skills. These principles can be applied to various learning outcomes, such as motor skills, intellectual skills, and cognitive strategies (Gagné and Briggs, 1974). In addition, they can be applied at different instructional levels, for example, in sequencing a course, a topic within that course, a lesson within that topic, or a component within that lesson. This theory would imply that a teaching improvement method should be organized according to the hierarchical levels of learning tasks.

The above principles are most applicable to teaching improvement methods that are designed to teach instructional skills or cognitive strategies, e.g., concept-based methods and microteaching. Examination of these methods for evidence of a subclassification of skills may provide insight into the method's potential effectiveness in teaching complex ideas or skills.

QUESTION 12: Is practice included as an integral component of the teaching-improvement method?

According to behaviorist theory, recitation and repeated practice lead to greater mastery and retention of material to be learned. Furthermore, it has been shown that distributed practice is better than massed practice; that is, if practice is spread over successive days rather than lumped into one session, it will result in more effective learning and retention. This principle is especially applicable to rote learned information, motor skill behavior (Brown and Herrnstein, 1975, p 122), and social skills (Trower et al., 1978, pp 71—72). Since many teaching behaviors may be seen as complex social skills, this theory would imply that practice is important in the acquisition of teaching behaviors.

Residents may not master important teaching skills (e.g., questioning, providing feedback) by discovering them, by being told about them, or by observing them. Practice may be necessary.

QUESTION 13: Does the teaching improvement method include feedback regarding the residents' performance of the teaching behaviors being taught in the method?

Behaviorist theory lends support to the importance of feedback in the acquisition of knowledge and skills (Sahakian, 1984, p. 409). Theorists argue that it is critical for a person to receive information about the closeness of his actual performance to a predefined desired behavior. According to Bruner (1966, p 50) "Learning depends upon knowledge of results at a time when and at a place where the knowledge can be used for correction. Instruction increases the appropriate timing and placing of corrective knowledge." Based on trial and error learning in animals, it is recommended that feedback be given as close in time to the behavior as feasible. However, with respect to the learning of complex human skills such as teaching, this recommendation may need to be qualified. Some research suggests that feedback can be delayed and still be effective (Trower et al., 1978, pp. 72–74). Studies in microteaching (Brusling, 1974, pp 45-46) indicate that feedback delayed for days may be as effective as immediate feedback. Researchers suggest that delayed feedback may be desirable as a means of increasing the objectivity of the teacher who may become less defensive in his analysis of performance after a lapse of time. Thus, there is some variation possible as to the exact timing of feedback for acquiring complex teaching skills. However, the usefulness of feedback in acquiring a skill is clear.

QUESTION 14: If a method uses visual aids (diagrams, slides, videotapes, feedback from rating forms), is the presented information organized in space in such a way that resembles the conceptual organization of the information?

Gestalt Psychology Theories

The school of Gestalt psychology was developed in the early twentieth century around principles of "wholistic," organic perception. Gestalt psychologists devised ways to demonstrate the theory that the brain has built-in systems for organizing visual information. The premises of Gestalt theories have strongly influenced the modern theories of cognitive psychology. Gestalt psychologists have argued that the relationships among visual stimuli (i.e., proximity, similarity, and simplicity) trigger the brain to organize them. Principles from Gestalt theory have implications for instructional materials design. According to Gestalt principles, perceptual representations of visual material should highlight the essential features being taught (Bower and Hilgard, 1981, p. 543). This principle might seem most easily applicable to teaching improvement methods that emphasize the presentation of material, such as concept-based methods. However, it may also have relevance to other methods such as student feedback or peer evaluation. For example, when written feedback from evaluation forms is provided, is it presented in such a way as to highlight key issues?

QUESTION 15: Does the teaching-improvement method provide explanations of the bases and interrelationships among concepts taught or encourage the participants to discover them?

Another principle from Gestalt psychology states that an array of information is better retained and transferred when the learner understands reasons or principles underlying phenomena as opposed to rote memorization of material (Katona, 1940). How, for example, do phenomena fit together, what parts depend on or support others? Material is less likely to be forgotten when it is made meaningful and logically interconnected. In training residents, we are not attempting to impart a series of skills that are prescriptively used in given situations. Rather, resident education in teaching should impart general guidelines and principles as well as specific behaviors for use in fostering learning. Residents would then be able to use (1) their knowledge of general rules, (2) their own creativity, and (3) their knowledge of their students' needs to decide on appropriate teaching approaches.

With regard to teaching-improvement methods for residents, methods that neither (1) stimulate residents to develop a framework nor (2) provide a framework for understanding the basis for teaching behaviors may diminish retention of the behaviors and transference to the actual teaching setting. One might assume that a method providing opportunities for learner discussions or teacher presentations of general teaching principles (e.g., consultation with an educator, concept-based methods, seminars) would be most likely to assist residents. Other methods, such as student feedback or peer evaluation, have the potential to neglect this area unless the evaluation form is unique and organized by educational principles.

QUESTION 16: Does the teaching-improvement method incorporate educational strategies that assist residents in retention of information?

Cognitive Theory

Cognitive psychology attempts to understand the nature of human intelligence and how people think (Anderson, 1985, p. 11). Cognitive psychologists are interested in how sensory input is transformed, elaborated, stored, recovered, and used (Neisser, 1967, p. 4). Seeing, hearing, and remembering are seen as constructive acts. Basic human information processing systems include scanning and holding, solving problems, remembering, generating and classifying, and ordering and relating. In moving information from short- term to long-term storage, we code, group, reorganize, and analyze that information. These processes of rehearsal and reformulation of information serve as means of compensating for the limited capacity for simultaneous handling of items of information. They provide a way of elaborating material, making it more meaningful and related to known things (Brown and Herrnstein, 1975, p. 130). To help learners to remember material, teachers can encourage the use of the following techniques for recoding: (1) group the concepts to be learned into similar categories, (2) visualize mental images of previously presented material, and (3) create and rehearse meaningful sentences relating each concept to the others.

Any teaching improvement method may be seen as having important messages for a teacher to remember. For example, ratings from student or peer evaluations may highlight particular teacher strengths or problems that should be remembered and later addressed in teaching. Concept-based or skills training methods also have important specific goals. Therefore, it is appropriate to ask of any teaching improvement method whether it encourages learners to use techniques to enhance memory of important lessons.

QUESTION 17: Does the method present information in contexts of eventual use?

Research in cognitive psychology suggests that knowledge should be represented in a form appropriate to the way it will be used (Norman, 1982, p. 104). When general educational concepts or principles are presented in a teaching improvement method, the relevance of those concepts to the teaching roles of the participants should be made clear. The original conception of microteaching, in which teachers were to be faced with real teaching situations with real pupils, capitalized on this principle of having skills practiced in a setting similar to the setting of ultimate use. This principle is also applicable to teaching improvement methods for residents. It is important to examine whether the material used (e.g., rating forms) or the concepts or skills taught are relevant to the eventual teaching context for the resident.

QUESTION 18: Is modeling incorporated into the teaching improvement method?

Social Learning Theory

Social learning theorists argue that it is difficult to explain some changes in behavior without assuming that learning occurs as an internal cognitive event rather than through the direct experiences involved in actual performance; that is, learning may occur as a result of the thinking process rather than as a result of the behavioral experience. Observational learning, as part of Bandura's social learning model, extends the principles of conditioning to internal and unobservable processes such as thinking (Marx and Bunch, 1977, p 482). Social learning theory suggests that one can not only better understand, but also acquire, behaviors through modeling. Functionally, a model is defined as any stimulus array so organized that an observer can extract and act on the main information conveyed by environmental events without needing to first perform overtly (Rosenthal and Bandura, 1978, p. 622).

Although one might generally think of modeling as observing someone else perform a behavior on film or in person, Rosenthal and Bandura (1978) describe at least three levels of modeling: symbolic, vicarious, and participant. Symbolic, or covert, modeling is exemplified by a process such as cognitively visualizing, or thinking about, an episode without actually observing it performed. Vicarious modeling occurs when others are observed performing a desired behavior. Participant, or overt, modeling refers to participants actually performing a desired behavior. Although participant modeling, or practice, is usually considered the most helpful exercise, it is important to note that for some behaviors, symbolic or vicarious modeling is effective for performing the skill. The type of modeling necessary may depend on the complexity of the skill and the familiarity of the participants with the skill components. For the purposes of skill acquisition in a teaching improvement method, it would seem important to have modeling at some level (symbolic, vicarious, or participant) incorporated in the method.

CONCLUSIONS

In this chapter, we have presented several approaches to teaching improvement and discussed selected educational and psychological theories to assist educators in developing or selecting a teaching improvement method for residents. We have listed specific questions that could be asked about a method to assess the strength of its theoretical basis and possibly its likelihood of being effective.

It is critical to note that teaching improvement methods have not been empirically compared based on their incorporation of different theoretically based components. Therefore, it is impossible to state for a given set of teachers in a given instructional setting which of the theoretical guidelines are most important for a method's effectiveness. In addition, the choice of a method may depend on practical constraints of time or availability of trained personnel to conduct the methods. However, we hope that the theory-based questions will allow an educator not only to develop or select a teaching improvement method for residents on the basis of practical constraints, but also to choose an approach on theoretical grounds.

One could argue that the most effective methods would incorporate the greatest number of components. This may, in fact, be the basis for the effectiveness of the complex, multicomponent methods that have been developed. Nonetheless, we hope that this chapter does not simply lead the reader to conclude that the more complex a method is, the better. This would not be a useful approach for institutions that may not have adequate personnel to implement such methods. It may be that some components are more critical to the success of a method than others. We have proposed that analyzing these methods on theoretical grounds can provide insight into the basis for their effectiveness. Our further hope is that this chapter will promote research efforts to develop a thorough classification of teaching improvement approaches based on a theoretical framework. With such a classification, empirical comparisons of these methods on a theoretical basis can begin to answer not only the question of what components are most essential to an effective teaching improvement method, but more importantly, the question of why.

CHAPTER 7
Evaluating Resident Teaching

DAVID M. IRBY

Residents function in three interdependent roles: as clinicians, learners, and teachers. While carrying heavy patient-care loads, residents actively engage in learning the knowledge, skills, and attitudes needed to practice medicine successfully. In the midst of this fast-paced professional life, residents also provide most clinical instruction to both medical students and other residents.

The responsibility for evaluating these three roles rests with the faculty. In most residency training programs, performance expectations are outlined for clinical responsibilities and learning, and occasionally for teaching. Faculty members provide direct supervision, guided learning experiences, and evaluation so that residents are able to master their clinical and learning responsibilities. Traditionally, however, relatively little emphasis has been placed on residents' teaching abilities. A need exists both to assess and guide development of teaching competencies in a fashion similar to that provided for the development of clinical skills.

The instructional role of residents is a natural extension of their clinical responsibilities. Because of the resident's availability and proximity to medical students and other residents, learning takes place in informal as well as formal settings. Approximately 70% of clinical learning among medical students (and residents) is provided by house staff (Stenchever et al., 1979). Indeed, Weinholtz (Mattern et al., 1983) found that individual learning is closely associated with team learning.

To improve the quality of teaching by residents, an effective system for evaluating such teaching must be implemented. This requires that the purposes for evaluation be determined, criteria for evaluation be established, and policies and procedures be developed. This chapter describes how to create such a system and offers guidance on the design of instruments and procedures.

PURPOSES OF EVALUATION

The teaching abilities of residents should be assessed in order to improve their teaching, to certify the quality of teaching they provide, and to improve the overall residency program. The primary purpose for evaluating teaching should be to improve the quality of instruction. Residents, like other teachers, rarely receive feedback on their teaching and therefore lack the knowledge needed to improve their teaching skills. A systematic evaluation program can directly inform residents of their strengths and of areas to improve. With time, consistent feedback can be a powerful motivator for change.

Teaching should be part of the resident performance evaluation process. To certify that resident performance is satisfactory, each role must be assessed: clinician, learner, and teacher. Including teaching in the performance evaluation reinforces the importance of the teaching function.

To assess the overall quality of the residency program, information is also needed on teaching quality. Because residents provide most of the clinical instruction, these data can be used to assess the overall strengths and limitations of the residency training program.

The evaluation of teaching in any academic program should assess the teaching effectiveness of faculty as well. By giving equal consideration to faculty and residents, and by providing assistance to improve resident and faculty skills, the program can create an atmosphere that promotes teaching excellence and supports improvement efforts.

CRITERIA FOR TEACHING EXCELLENCE

When developing evaluation forms and procedures, items should be based on criteria identified in the literature as being associated with teaching effectiveness. I have identified several facets of teaching effectiveness that have emerged consistently from studies of classroom and clinical teaching (Irby, 1978a, b; Irby and Rakestraw, 1981). Four factors are required for effective classroom and clinical teaching: (1)

knowledge and analytical ability, (2) organization and clarity of presentation, (3) enthusiasm and stimulation of interest, and (4) group-instructional skills. Three additional factors unique to clinical instruction include (5) clinical-supervisory skills, (6) clinical competence, and (7) positive professional characteristics. Rating schemes based on these factors might include the following instructional abilities:

Instructor knowledge: discusses current developments, shows that he reads broadly, discusses divergent points of view, relates topics to other disciplines, and directs students/residents to useful literature in the field.

Organization and clarity of presentation: explains clearly, presents material in an organized manner, summarizes, emphasizes what is important, and communicates what is expected to be learned.

Enthusiasm and stimulation of interest: shows dynamism and energy, enjoys teaching, and has an interesting style of presentation that stimulates interest in the subject.

Group instructional skills: encourages active participation, establishes rapport, shows respect for and personal interest in students/residents, listens attentively, and questions students/residents in a nonthreatening manner.

Clinical competence: objectively defines and synthesizes patient problems, demonstrates skill at data-gathering and problem-solving, and maintains rapport with patients.

Clinical supervision: observes student/resident performance frequently, identifies learner strengths and limitations objectively, provides personal and professional support, and offers feedback and positive reinforcement.

Professional characteristics: is self-critical, takes responsibility, recognizes own limitations, does not appear to be arrogant, shows sensitivity and respect for others.

Other facets of teaching effectiveness that appear less frequently in the literature include challenge and high expectations, fairness, and level of difficulty in evaluation and grading.

EVALUATION STRATEGIES

Teaching can be evaluated in several ways, characterized under these strategies: rating forms completed by learners, observational methods, peer review, and self-assessment.

Student-rating forms can be used to collect information from both medical students and residents. Such quantitative measures of teaching performance should be collected systematically in both classroom and clinical settings. Learners know whether or not they are learning and therefore are in a unique position to comment on such qualities as the resident's organization and clarity of presentation, enthusiasm, and instructional skills. These ratings data are relatively inexpensive to obtain and have been found to be both valid and reliable (Feldman, 1976; Irby and Rakestraw, 1981).

A substantial amount of research done on student ratings of teaching in higher education has led to the following conclusions:

Learners are able to make reliable and consistent judgments about the instructor and the instruction offered, both within a class and across time. Correlations among raters typically range from .70 to .90 (Aleamoni, 1981;Costin et al., 1971; Feldman, 1976; Irby and Rakestraw, 1981).

Learners are able to evaluate accurately different aspects of teacher performance (for example, enthusiasm, teaching methods, course content) and thus qualify as discriminating judges (Aleamoni, 1981; Costin et al., 1971; Feldman, 1976; Irby, 1978; Irby and Rakestraw, 1981).

Ratings on a given instructor are consistent over time; alumni ratings of faculty are consistent with current student ratings of the same faculty member (Aleamoni, 1981; Marsh and Overall, 1979).

The validity of student-rating forms is substantiated by the judgment of experts and by earlier research, which ensures that the rating scales reflect the most important aspects of instruction (Costin et al., 1971). Further evidence of validity comes from studies that have correlated student ratings with other indicators of teaching competence, for example: peer ratings, expert judges' ratings, alumni ratings, and student learning. Moderate-to-high positive correlations were found in 4 studies reviewed by Aleamoni and Hexner (1980).

Thus, learner ratings of instruction have been found to be valid and reliable measures of teaching effectiveness. Such quantitative measures of teaching are easy to design, administer, and analyze and should be used systematically.

At the University of Washington School of Medicine a rating form has been developed to assess clinical teaching effectiveness of both residents and faculty members. A noncomputerized version of the form is found in Appendix I at the end of this volume. This rating form is administered at the end of each rotation and the results are summarized semiannually or annually. Each resident and faculty member receives a summary report of ratings and his teaching, along with the average rating of all faculty, for each item. The reports are often given out at workshops designed to improve teaching.

For resident leadership of conferences and more group-oriented classroom teaching, a short rating form can be used. This can be as simple as a three-by-five card with an overall rating for the session to be written at the top of one side, and comments on strengths to be given below the overall rating. On the other side comments can be written regarding recommendations for improvement. The cards can then be collected and given to the resident at the conclusion of the conference.

In addition to learner perceptions of teaching, observational methods for assessing teaching are also available. These methods include participant-observer descriptions of teaching, the use of audiotape and videotape, and expert consultant observation. The key to effective observational methods is to define clearly the criteria for evaluation in advance. From the criteria of teaching effectiveness described above, several peer-observation forms were developed to focus observer attention on the instructional aspects of teaching. (See Appendixes II and III.)

When using audiotape and videotape for evaluation and improvement of resident teaching, clear expectations for the use of the tape medium should be established in advance. The residents could review the tape on their own and evaluate the interchange before discussing it with peers, faculty, or educational consultants. Alternatively, someone could review the audiotape with the resident and discuss each part of it with him or her. The peer review form can be helpful in identifying both the strengths and the weaknesses of the instructional event.

For faculty, peer review of teaching is a well-established, although infrequently used, method for evaluating and improving teaching. This mechanism may also be used to review teaching of residents. One of the chief resident's responsibilities can be to provide feedback to the junior residents on their teaching abilities. Chief residents or faculty can convene residents periodically (monthly, quarterly, semiannually) to discuss the teaching quality and contributions of each resident. The structure for these meetings should enable the participants to identify the strengths of each person involved and to recommend means by which that person could improve. The positive and supportive nature of this structure should be monitored carefully. Residents may be more comfortable in such a setting if faculty members are not present. Leadership for these peer-review sessions needs to be carefully structured, however, so that the chief resident (or person designated) can facilitate this interchange in a positive and constructive manner.

Self assessment is another method of evaluating teaching. A Self-Assessment Inventory for Clinical and Classroom Teaching in Medicine has been helpful to faculty and residents in assessing their own teaching abilities (see Appendix IV). The inventory lists 54 teacher behaviors clustered under seven factors of teaching effectiveness. The form is useful in identifying specific areas for improvement and specific areas of strength on which to build. It has been used most frequently in workshop settings and as a part of a personal consultation process.

Faculty should consistently monitor resident teaching, just as they review resident clinical competence and learning. An item related to teaching contributions should be incorporated into the attending rating forms for clinical performance of residents. This item will enable faculty members to comment on the general and particular teaching contributions of residents.

GUIDELINES FOR RATING FORMS

When designing rating forms for use in the clinical-teaching arena, the following guidelines may be helpful:

1. Select items for the rating form that reflect the characteristics of teaching effectiveness identified in the literature; for example being knowledgeable and analytical, being enthusiastic and stimulating, interacting skillfully with learners, establishing rapport, providing direction and feedback, being accessible, and demonstrating overall quality in teaching. A similar set of items should be used on all forms.
2. Use the same rating scale on all forms, for example, excellent, very good, good, fair, poor. A seven-point scale also works well. Provide an option for *Not Observed* or *Not Applicable* as well.
3. State directions clearly and concisely on the forms.
4. Provide space for comments that list strengths and recommendations for improvement. By soliciting positive and constructive

comments, the evaluation encourages residents to respond affirmatively to suggestions for improvement.

5. Limit the form to a single page, when possible, to reduce writer fatigue and to provide better quality comments and ratings. In clinical teaching, where students/residents are exposed to multiple residents and faculty, a one-page form that rates several residents/teachers works most effectively. Appendix I is an example.

MANAGEMENT OF EVALUATION

Administering an evaluation system can be facilitated by adopting the following suggestions. First, hand out rating forms in group settings where possible. Make it easy for respondents to complete the evaluation forms. Use the last 5 minutes of a conference, grand rounds, or a class to distribute the forms, and ask the residents/students to complete them before leaving. This will increase student/resident willingness to give feedback and will improve the response rate.

To assess teaching effectiveness successfully in clinical settings, a systematic data-collection procedure is needed. Someone must be designated as being responsible for ensuring that the rating forms are distributed, collected, and tabulated, and the results shared with the residents. The ratings should be summarized and given to the residents at predetermined intervals (for example, semiannually or annually).

Residency directors can use information from a teaching evaluation to support their own observations of the resident's overall performance. When the director meets with each resident for periodic performance review, the director can provide specific feedback, explore problems identified by the evaluation, and develop improvement strategies with the resident. Excellent residents may need only positive reinforcement while poor performers may require more thorough assessment, counseling, and support.

The setting in which teaching-evaluation summaries are returned to residents can have a significant impact on resident receptivity to suggestions made for improvement and to the system as a whole. Combining teaching improvement activities with the sharing of results from teaching evaluations can set a positive tone for the entire process. Presentations on clinical teaching skills by faculty or educational consultants, when combined with group discussion and role plays, provide residents with helpful tools for improving their teaching (Skeff, 1983; Skeff et al., 1984) Most residents are grateful to receive this form of assistance. A half-day workshop that included a meal proved successful for this kind of evaluation–improvement effort (Irby et al., 1982).

Summarizing and reporting results of teaching evaluation can be tedious and time-consuming. Consideration should be given to computerizing the scoring and reporting process. For a minimal initial investment, rating forms can be optically scanned and reports generated by microcomputers. This process reduces the burdensome task of collation and report generation.

The result of all this evaluation of teaching performance should be to reward teaching excellence among residents, improve resident training, and ultimately enhance patient care. The information can be incorporated into the overall evaluation of a resident to facilitate positive reinforcement of this important aspect of professional responsibility. Teaching awards and other forms of recognition can also create a climate of interest and excitement about teaching.

IMPACT OF TEACHING EVALUATION

Feedback from learner ratings and peer review of teaching can serve as an impetus for changing teaching practices, particularly if specific improvements are suggested. Studies show that faculty teaching changes most when student ratings provide new information to the faculty member, when the ratings are at variance with the teacher's self-assessment, and when consultation is provided. In a review of the literature, Levinson-Rose and Menges (1981) concluded that feedback from student ratings leads to improvement, especially when supplemented with consultation. Student ratings of clinical teaching, when combined with semiannual department faculty workshops, have decidedly improved teaching (Irby et al., 1982).

Evaluation of teaching within a residency program should be an integral part of the overall academic program (and faculty should be evaluated as well). Information collected on teaching should be incorporated into resident performance evaluation as one of the three major performance areas (patient care, learning, and teaching). The information derived from evaluation should stimulate, guide, and maintain behavioral change in resident teaching.

CHAPTER 8

How Clinical Teaching Is Studied

DONN WEINHOLTZ

Clinical teaching, like many forms of teaching, is an art. The characteristics that make it an art are the very things that make the scientific study of clinical teaching an intriguing and demanding process. What are these artistic characteristics? Gage (1984) has described them well.

> Teaching is an instrumental or practical art, not a fine art aimed at creating beauty for its own sake. As an instrumental art, teaching is something that departs from recipes, formulas, or algorithms. It requires improvisation; spontaneity; the handling of hosts of considerations of form, style, pace, rhythm, and appropriateness . . .

Teaching's artistic quality is especially apparent in clinical teaching. Occurring as it does in work settings, clinical teaching places a maximum demand on the instructor's ability to respond to events encountered daily and to use these events for promoting learning. Given such a type of teaching, Gage's (1984) caveat against trying to reduce effective teaching to systematic formulas or algorithms deserves special heed.

Researchers studying clinical teaching must find ways of capturing the richness of such teaching while isolating those particular aspects that are associated with predictable outcomes. For such research to be of any real value it must be converted for use by clinical teachers. The results should find their way back to clinical teachers and help those teachers to enhance their art.

METHODS OF STUDYING TEACHING

The research studies investigating clinical teaching can, like the research studies in other scientific endeavors, be separated into three broad categories: (1) descriptive, (2) correlational, and (3) experimental. Descriptive studies are conducted using either qualitative techniques (e.g., participant observation or interview) or quantitative techniques (e.g., numerically scored survey) in order to isolate key variables. Correlational studies are conducted to quantify the strength of the relationships between variables. Experimental studies are conducted to determine if causal relationships exist between variables, and if manipulation of one variable (or set of variables) yields changes in another variable (or set of variables).

Much of the clinical teaching research has been descriptive. It has focused on identifying key variables of interest while leading only to speculation on possible causal relationships between teaching behaviors and specific outcomes experienced by learners. For example, in frequently cited studies Stritter et al. (1975) and Irby (1978a) factor analyzed data solicited from medical students in order to generate general dimensions of effective clinical teaching. These studies, conducted independently, yielded complementary general findings. Stritter et al. (1975) found that effective clinical teachers: (1) provide a personal environment in which the student is an active participant; (2) maintain a positive attitude toward teaching and students; (3) concentrate on the clinical problem solving process rather than factual material alone; (4) use student centered instructional strategies; (5) demonstrate a humanistic orientation in their interactions with patients and students; and (6) emphasize references and research findings. Irby (1978a) found that clinical teachers demonstrate: (1) organization and clarity; (2) group instructional skill; (3) enthusiasm and stimulation; (4) knowledge; (5) clinical supervision; (6) clinical competence; and (7) professional characteristics.

Another set of descriptive studies, relying primarily on observations of clinical teaching, yielded some findings consistent with the two survey studies just mentioned, several provided more detailed accounts regarding obstacles to clinical teaching in specific settings such as attending rounds and work rounds (Daggett, 1977; Foley and Smilansky, 1979; Hinz, 1966; Jason, 1962; Mattern et al., 1983; Maxwell et al., 1983;

Payson and Barchas, 1965; Reichsman et al., 1964; Tremonti and Biddle, 1982; and Weinholtz, 1981). Although these studies helped to clarify some of the unique aspects of medical clinical teaching, they only suggested possible quantifiable relationships between clinical teaching and learner performance. Nevertheless, these studies made it clear that clinical instruction on hospital wards is a group phenomenon in which all the physicians, and other health professionals on the medical service team, play substantial roles.

Among the physicians on the team, the attending physician assumes the difficult teak of providing teaching and patient-care leadership to medical students and house staff who often view the attending physician as an outsider on the ward. The intimidating nature of the attending physician's role often causes the attending physician to focus on what the attending physician perceives the interns want: detailed medical information. Often the attending physician can only provide this detail in his subspecialization area, and the attending physician tends to overemphasize the subspeciality, neglecting more general medical content and psychosocial issues.

The ward resident occupies the team position between the interns and students on one hand and the attending physician on the other. The resident is the ward manager who is expected to facilitate attending rounds in cooperation with the attending physician. Too often the manner in which the attending physician expects the resident to accomplish this task is not clearly defined, and the resident simply "wings it" according to his perceptions of the whims and capabilities of the attending physician. Attending physicians and residents may experience confusion and frustration in this sort of relationship.

The interns, especially early in their internships, are frequently overwhelmed by their patient-care responsibilities. Eager to obtain the medical knowledge necessary for dealing with their patients' immediate problems, the interns actively pursue what they perceive as immediately useful, and become frustrated when diverted from that course. Their concentration on getting the "right medical answers" often causes them to lose sight of important psychosocial patient-management issues.

Medical students, the lowest ranking "physicians" on the team, thrive on their hard-earned exposure to real clinical experiences, but grow tired of performing routine functions ("scutwork") on the wards. Craving new experiences and responsibilities, students often complain about being overlooked by the housestaff and intimidated by attending physicians. Feeling as though they are not in a powerful enough position to take the initiative regarding their learning, many students slip into passive roles.

Within this challenging team context there are an unlimited number of ways for attending physicians and residents to design and implement instructional experiences. Recently, clinical teaching researchers have begun conducting correlational and experimental studies to assess the impact of certain instructional approaches (Edwards et al., 1985; Jewett et al., 1982; Petzel et al., 1982; Skeff, 1983; Skeff and Stratos, 1985; Skeff et al., 1985; Weinholtz et al., 1985a, 1986a). In the correlational studies, the researchers have been investigating the strength of the relationships between teaching and various measures such as ratings of learner performance, self-reports of learning, and learner ratings of teaching effectiveness. In the experimental studies, the researchers have been attempting to discover whether changes in teaching yield predictable changes in the types of measures previously described.

To date, the correlational and experimental studies have demonstrated that clinical teachers who adopt similar instructional approaches to those advocated by Stritter et al. (1975) and Irby (1978a) appear to positively impact on students' subsequent clinical performances (Petzel et al., 1982) and students' assessments of their learning (Skeff, 1983). Instructional workshops, seminars, or individualized consultations have been shown to have a positive impact on clinical teachers' attitudes (Edwards et al., 1985; Skeff, 1983; Skeff and Stratos, 1985), medical students' ratings of clinical teachers (Edwards et al., 1985) and clinical teachers' behaviors (Skeff, 1983; Skeff and Stratos, 1985). Finally, my colleagues and I (Weinholtz et al., 1986a) have shown that the impact of certain clinical teachers' behaviors (e.g., questioning and evaluating) on learner ratings of teaching effectiveness tends to vary with the level of learner (i.e., student, intern, or resident), context of behavior (e.g., patient presentation and discussion, patient interview, and patient examination), and location of behavior (i.e., conference room, hallway, bedside).

This shift toward correlational studies and experimentation is encouraging. Research on clinical teaching is now apparently completing its initial descriptive-correlational-experimental cycle (Rosenshine and Furst, 1973). Preliminary findings have been described. The strengths of some of the relationships suggested by those findings have either been confirmed or brought into question. Finally, experiments have been conducted to examine the usefulness of the findings for clinical teachers.

PROPOSALS FOR THREE STUDIES OF RESIDENTS' CLINICAL TEACHING

Three hypothetical studies of residents' clinical teaching clearly do not exhaust the full range of research possibilities regarding such teaching.

They do, however, show one potential way for implementing a descriptive-correlational-experimental cycle.

All good research is time-consuming, and these three studies (or their reasonable facsimiles) necessitate substantial time commitments by the participating researchers. To the extent that clinical faculty or residents wishing to conduct such educational research find the time constraints incompatible with their busy clinical schedules, seeking collaborative relationships with educational researchers interested in investigating issues in medical education is advisable. Stritter (1983) has described the following benefits of such team efforts for participating health professionals: (1) increasing awareness of educational issues; (2) developing social science research skills; and (3) initiating a line of related projects leading to publications and presentations.

I have found that periodically reviewing findings with selected persons not engaged in the data collection is beneficial. Such persons can play devil's advocates, challenging the researchers' assumptions whenever possible, or they can act as interpreters, offering their insights regarding the phenomena described by the researchers. These roles might well be adopted by busy clinical faculty interested in promoting and coordinating participant observation research, but unable to engage in the fieldwork themselves. The roles of fieldworkers, on the other hand, might be adopted by either seasoned educational researchers or education graduate students.

The studies described here address clinical teaching by residents on general internal medicine wards. The focus is thus on the teaching done by residents on inpatient services as opposed to that done in ambulatory care settings. The first two studies address this general research question: What is effective clinical teaching by residents? The third study addresses this question: Can residents' clinical teaching effectiveness be enhanced through participation in a teaching-improvement program? This second question has already been investigated (Edwards et al., 1985), but the suppositions in Edwards' research regarding effective teaching have been drawn from general principles of instruction (Gagne, 1977) and the logical adaptation of these principles to clinical settings (Stritter and Flair, 1980).

Although such suppositions may indeed be valid, it is possible that there are unique features of residents' clinical teaching, as yet not understood, that might affect recommendations derived from general instructional principles. The purpose of the first two studies is to discover (Study 1) and validate (Study 2) such features. Because Study 2 and Study 3 flow directly from Study 1, and because the goal of Study 1 is the discovery of unknown features, the descriptions of the studies, especially of the second and third, must be somewhat tentative and not too prescriptive. General recommendations for design and method are all that will be provided. These recommendations will approximate those published recently (Weinholtz et al., 1985a and Weinholtz and Friedman, 1985b) for the study of clinical teaching by attending physicians. Although such studies could easily be conducted at any major, university-affiliated teaching hospital, for heuristic purposes, we will assume that the studies would be conducted at the University of Iowa's University Hospital and the Veterans Administration Hospital close to the University of Iowa.

Study 1: Description Through Participant Observation

To discover features about residents' clinical teaching that might affect generally accepted recommendations regarding effective clinical teaching, the preferred method is participant observation. Such observation does not bind researchers to prejudgments about a problem. It combines a variety of flexible data-gathering approaches, and frees investigators to apply what they learn throughout the entire research process. Participant observation enables investigators to link statements and actions of those involved in the study. Furthermore the method places researchers "... in a better position to impute motives from observations, to pace observations ... and to incorporate what may have first appeared to be irrelevant data into subsequent analysis" (Denzin, 1978, p. 212).

Although participant observation research is subject to substantial threats to internal and external validity—via subjectivity predominating in validation—such threats can be minimized through careful planning and implementation (McCall and Simmons, 1969; Weinholtz, 1981). For an exceptionally clear and practical description of how to conduct participant observation studies, the reader should consult Lofland (1971). In particular, Lofland provides excellent guidelines for recording and analyzing field materials from observations and interviews, the two primary methods of participant observation research.

One great challenge facing participant observation researchers, or any researchers using qualitative techniques, is to interpret emprirical findings observed in natural settings without bias or preordination. For example, to the extent that researchers conducting a study might focus disproportionately on the recommendations of Gagne (1977) and Stritter and Flair (1980), or any additional theoretical orientation to empirical findings, the researchers might be oblivious to unexpected, but important, events. Obviously, this dilemma is not absolutely resolvable because human beings inevitably select perceptions. Nevertheless, one can take certain steps to overcome selective perception, while clearly articulating the researchers' orientations for the benefit of other investigators.

Pertinent recommendations have been implemented and explained by Weinholtz and Friedman (1985b). Although addressing these recommendations in detail would be beyond our need here, those general procedures offered will be used to illustrate the primary phases of Study 1.

The general phases which Charles Friedman and I (Weinholtz and Friedman, 1985b) have suggested are:

1. Prospectively determine the framework of the study: goals, setting, sampling procedures, and data-collection techniques.
2. Before starting the study, review the theoretical empirical literature assumed to be most pertinent to the interpretation of the phenomena under investigation. State broad, preliminary assumptions derived from this review and any orienting concepts that seem useful to the structure of the study.
3. Conduct a pilot phase of the study, using the techniques chosen for fieldwork. Follow up the pilot phase with a several-week respite from fieldwork, during which theoretical perspectives and focused assumptions emerging from the pilot phase are stated.
4. Complete the fieldwork, refining interpretations incrementally, and prepare a final report giving the key results of the study, preferably also including a set of propositions for further investigation. Each phase is discussed as recommendations for the initial study are described.

Phase 1: Determine the Study Framework

The primary goal of this study is to develop criteria for discriminating effective from ineffective teaching by residents on general internal medicine wards. The settings of the study are the five general internal medicine wards of the University of Iowa Hospital and the four general internal medicine wards of the Veterans Administration Hospital staffed by University of Iowa faculty, housestaff, and medical students. During the year, these nine wards provide opportunities to observe 108 different medical service teams as they engage in patient care, teaching, and learning. As with most general internal medicine services, the wards in this study are staffed by teams generally consisting of a single attending physician, a second-year or third-year resident, two or three first-year residents and two or three medical students.

For this study 18 different teams, 2 from each of the nine wards, will be observed for 2 weeks apiece (6 days per week) during a 9-month period. With involvement of 18 teams the study will guarantee observations of about 72 residents: 18 second-year or third-year residents and 54 first-year residents. The participant observation research will be conducted by 2 field workers, each observing a separate team during the same month. The ward teams will be chosen at random, without replacement, until each of the wards has been observed twice during the 9 months. Teams will be observed on the first and third weeks of their month of ward duty. Intervening weeks will be used by the field workers to compile and compare field materials and discuss with each other findings and interpretations. Central to the discussions will be the emerging focus of the study with regard to the theoretical and empirical literature used to interpret the study's findings.

The decisions presented here on the number of fieldworkers, number of teams observed, and length and time of observations were arbitrarily chosen from a seemingly endless number of possibilities. The choices offer a reasonably extensive sample of resident teaching behaviors, across a number of key settings, by different residents, at different times of the year, viewed and interpreted by different observers. Researchers proposing studies at other institutions would naturally have to decide what would be appropriate based on the particular constraints and resources confronting them. Maxwell et al. (1983) and I (Weinholtz, 1981) have described participant-observation studies using different numbers of field workers and different numerical and temporal sampling patterns. The guidelines provided here are merely suggestive of the many intriguing possiblities available.

As one enters the study, the types of data to be collected by the field workers must be addressed. Considerations must include the periods during which observations will take place, the types of interviews that will be conducted in conjunction with the observations (e.g., informal-brief-untaped or systematic-extensive-audiotaped), and whether or not any documents (e.g., evaluation forms completed by residents on medical students, or vice versa) will be reviewed in conjunction with the observations and interviews.

For this study, each observer will follow each ward resident, on the first six teams observed, for most of one working day (e.g., 8:00 AM—6:00 PM) to discover when the residents engage in teaching activities. While extremely time consuming, such observations will enable the observers to determine whether teaching is generally restricted to formal occasions, such as morning work rounds, attending rounds, x-ray rounds, and any other scheduled conferences, or whether teaching is more likely to occur in informal, unscheduled sessions spontaneously developing throughout the day. After the first 4 days of observations for each of these first six teams, the fieldworkers will determine a strategy for further observing each team. For example, after the four residents on Team 1 are observed, for 1 day apiece, the fieldworker assigned to that team will decide how to allot the observational time for the remain ing 8 days of observations. Because day-long observations tend to tire observers, the fieldworkers will decide on strategies designed to give them a respite from observations to engage in reflection time and to develop and organize field notes. One possible strategy would involve using the first 4 of the 8 remaining days strictly for observing all struc tured sessions (e.g., work rounds, attending rounds), and using the final 4 days for observing each of the four residents during "unstructured" time to observe spontaneous teaching opportunities that arise. After the first six teams are observed (three by each fieldworker), the field-workers can then decide whether or not the practice of reserving the first 4 days of the observation period for full-day observations should be retained, or whether it should be jettisoned in favor of some 2-week version of the lighter observation schedules.

Regarding the types of interviews to be conducted in the study, extended audiotaped interviews lasting about 1 hour will be conducted with each resident. These interviews (conducted after the 2 weeks of ob servations) will address the residents' perceptions of their own teaching, including their teaching of medical students, their peers, and even (in the case of senior residents) their attending physicians. The interviews will be conducted by the fieldworkers using an interviewing guide (i.e., a list of pertinent topics to be addressed) constructed by the field workers and the other study designers to ensure that all major concerns are addressed. In addition to these systematic interviews with the residents, the field workers will conduct brief, informal interviews with medical students and attending physicians at opportune moments during the 2 weeks of observations. These brief interviews, recorded by the field workers through jotted notes updated and enhanced later each day, will provide indications of how the residents' teaching is perceived by nonresident team members.

Two types of documents will be reviewed in conjunction with this study. First to be examined will be all written materials given to team members (i.e., students, residents, and attending physicians) by the Department of Internal Medicine, detailing the department's expectations regarding teaching and learning on clinical services. Reviewing these documents will determine the extent to which actual teaching practices conform with, or vary from, the official departmental communications. Second, the evaluations completed by team members at the end of their month on their services will be reviewed to determine whether team members' written comments on their teaching and learning experiences conform with their verbal comments to the fieldworkers. Qualitative comments on the evaluation forms may also provide an additional source of information on events occurring on the wards but not witnessed by the fieldworkers.

The final consideration in determining the overall framework of the study is deciding on procedures for recording, filing, and analyzing field materials. A variety of approaches might be adopted as to the recording of field notes, but such notes must be compiled and organized so as to yield a set of files that can be thoroughly and efficiently analyzed. The results of the study can then be interpreted. Lofland (1971) describes procedures for recording field notes and for development of multiple types of files. Those recommendations will be adopted in this study.

Phase 2: Derive Preliminary Assumptions and Orienting Concepts from the Literature

Although Phase 1 includes many crucial choices, the decisions made during that phase are relatively clear-cut compared with the decisions qualitative researchers must make to ground studies in the theoretical and research literature. The latter must guard against overly restricting their interpretations of unfolding events. The preliminary assumptions and orienting concepts necessary to provide some essential focus as field work begins will derive from two lines of clinical teaching literature: (1) studies evolving from the work of Gagné (1977) (including the publications of Stritter and Flair, 1980; Edwards et al., 1985; and Skeff et al., 1985) and (2) studies evolving from a group dynamics and leadership perspective (as illustrated by Weinholtz, 1981; Mattern et al. 1983; Weinholtz et al. 1985a). To the extent that these two lines of work clearly intersect, they would seem to do so in the "Experiential Development Model" described by me (Weinholtz, 1981) and my colleagues (Weinholtz et al., 1985c). Guidelines for stating initial assumptions and orienting concepts have been published (Weinholtz and Friedman, 1985b). The initial assumptions and orienting concepts should be sufficiently general to enable incorporation and varying interpretations of the variety of events likely to be witnessed in the field. The "Experiential Development Model" seems to meet these criteria, but its potentially biasing effect should be challenged regularly by the fieldworkers as they proceed through the next phase of the study.

Phase 3: Identify Theoretical Perspectives and Focused Assumptions after the Pilot Phase

As described in the framework of the study (Phase 1), observations of the first six teams conducted by the fieldworkers (three by each fieldworker) will involve one day-long observation of each resident on the six teams. When the observations (2 weeks per team) for these six teams are completed, the field workers will take a respite from their observational activities, and the pilot phase of the study will be considered finished. The pilot phase allows for the initial gathering of field materials within a loosely structured theoretical focus. The respite after the pilot phase permits the field workers and any other collaborators (e.g., participating clinical faculty members) to examine the findings from the pilot phase; to select additional theoretical and empirical perspectives to further guide the study (thus, narrowing the focus of the study); and to plot strategy regarding guidelines for future field work.

During preliminary planning stages it is impossible to preordain in any specific sense what will be said during the discussions immediately after the pilot phase. Still, certain topics clearly must be discussed. Among these will be the value of retaining day-long observations of individual residents and focusing more or less on either structured sessions (e.g., work rounds) or on other times of the day when spontaneous, one-on-one teaching is likely to occur. Another likely topic for discussion will be the extent to which the field workers should focus on the teaching of particular groups by different levels of residents: for example, medical students by first-year residents, versus medical students by third-year residents, versus first-year residents by third-year residents, versus attending physicians by third-year residents, versus patients by either level of resident. Finally, the discussions must address the extent to which the focus of the study can beneficially be narrowed and interpreted in conjunction with insights derived from the clinical teaching literature. For example, virtually any of the references from the clinical teaching literature cited in this volume might offer valuable insights for guiding the remainder of the study. Similarly, some previously unforeseen body of literature might be considered to provide valuable perspectives after consideration of certain events encountered during the pilot phase. For example, role theory or decision-making theory might come into play.

Whatever emerges during this phase, the discussions among the participating researchers must be wide-ranging and freewheeling before any particular directions are determined. The fieldworkers and their collaborators must critically challenge each other's assumptions and intepretations. Such discussions are no place for groupthink. Consensus must eventually emerge, but only after many perspectives have been aired.

Phase 4: Complete Field Work and Prepare Final Report

During the remainder of the field work and the compilation of the final report, the research team will work on refining the insights obtained during the pilot phase into a set of propositions suitable for confirmation or refutation through further research studies. These final propositions will be substantially more concrete than the stated assumptions developed during the preliminary stages of the study, and they should be stated in a manner clearly communicating suspected causal relationships among key variables. The formulation of the final propositions must involve the careful scrutiny of all field materials and all interpretations of those materials. To ensure their accuracy and preci sion, the final propositions should be rigorously challenged from many angles by the members of the collaborative research team (examples of such propositions are included in Weinholtz, 1981; and Weinholtz and Friedman, 1985b).

To conclude the discussion of this first study, a few comments are necessary. Again, the study described above is only one version of many possible similar studies that might be conducted. In spite of some very good research on residents' teaching during work rounds (Wilkerson, Lesky, and Medio, 1986), this sort of extensive qualitative study of residents' teaching has not been done. Ultimately, at least one such study must be conducted if the research on residents' teaching is to progress soundly. Preferably, several such qualitative case studies will be conducted, varying in their durations and their particular theoretical perspectives. These studies might yield findings suitable for the construction of descriptive surveys, further clarifying key variables. Then the common findings from these several studies can be summarized and additional studies can be designed to replicate or refute the findings. Similarly, the unique findings of individual studies can also be designated for further descriptive study. Such qualitative research will not authoritatively answer all the questions regarding effective teaching by residents; but it will begin to answer some, while ensuring that many more insightful questions are raised. From such questions, sound quantitative research emerges.

Study 2: Correlating Teaching Behaviors with Learner Ratings of Teaching Effectiveness

Several, but not necessarily all, of the propositions generated in the first study will likely address the relationship between particular teaching behaviors practiced by residents and learning outcomes experienced by other team members (e.g., medical students) or by patients. Although excellent for discovering relationships, qualitative studies are not best suited for convincingly demonstrating that those relationships truly do exist. For that purpose quantitative research methods are desirable, and correlational studies investigating the strength of the relationship between particular teaching behaviors and specified learning outcomes are the studies of choice. Such correlational studies may evolve as the logical extension of a descriptive study similar to that previously described, or they may be designed without the benefit of such studies. For example, an excellent correlational study of attending physician clinical teaching, begun without reliance on their own preliminary descriptive study, was conducted by Skeff et al. (1985). We (Weinholtz et al., 1986a), on the other hand, proceeded with a correlational study immediately after a descriptive study similar to that described in this chapter. Having different researchers converging on similar problems from slightly different perspectives is desirable. The extent to which such studies yield consistent findings enhances confidence in these findings. The extent to which findings differ raises important questions as to why they differ and what further research may be needed.

In any study examining the correlation of resident teaching behaviors with learning outcomes, several questions emerge as crucial within the study design. These questions address issues such as: (1) Which residents will be observed? (2) What instructional activities will be observed and how long will the observations take place? (3) Will observations be live, videotaped, or audiotaped events? (4) What particular instructional behaviors will be observed, and what type of instrument and recording mechanisms will be used to record those behaviors? (5) What measures of outcome will be adopted for correlation with the teaching behaviors? (6) Will any additional information be collected to supplement the outcome data? (7) How will the data collected in the study be managed, analyzed, and interpreted? These questions need to be addressed, but not necessarily in the order presented here.

As with Study 1, Study 2 reflects many arbitrary decisions necessary to provide an illustrative example. Many alternative correlational studies offer viable options, and if you want to conduct your own correlational studies, you should pursue the options perceived to be the most sound, given your particular research questions, resources, and constraints. The variables of Study 2 will be addressed in response to each of the questions listed above.

QUESTION 1: Which Residents Will Be Observed?

Any researcher hoping to conduct a study of teaching by residents that involves the observation and the recording of teaching behaviors and the correlation of these teaching behaviors with pertinent outcome measures immediately confronts a dilemma: Residents function at different levels and all engage in teaching. On whose teaching shall the study focus?

In this study, the focus will be on the third-year resident designated as the ward resident in charge of the medical service. He is the resident next in line to the attending physician in the service's chain of command. On occasion, two residents share this role. If such a situation is encountered, no observations will be recorded, due to the difficulty of observing and recording two residents' behaviors. Another service with a single resident serving as ward manager will be chosen instead.

The rationale for choosing to focus on this "senior" resident (or senior among the residents in the case of a second-year resident) is based on these premises: (1) records of teaching behavior are likely to be most accurate and reliable if the teaching of a single resident in a team situation is recorded by an observer, and (2) the senior resident's teaching is of particular interest because he has the greatest number of teaching responsibilities. The rationale for these premises will unfold more clearly in response to succeeding questions.

Resolving the issue of which level of resident to observe does not resolve the issue of how many "senior" residents should be observed. For this study, 27 third-year residents will be monitored by a single observer. This is the full contingent of third-year residents found in the Department of Internal Medicine at the University of Iowa. These ward residents will be observed as they teach on general internal medicine wards, the same wards involved in Study 1.

QUESTION 2: What Instructional Activities Will Be Observed, and For How Long a Time Will the Observations Take Place?

Although the preliminary descriptive study may have yielded many instructional activities engaged in by residents, this correlational study will focus on the teaching done by residents during morning work rounds. The rationale for the choice of work rounds rests on two primary factors: (1) morning work rounds are a regularly scheduled event occurring during a discrete portion of the day, and they are therefore readily observable; and (2) morning work rounds provide residents with many teaching opportunities during which they do not have to compete with attending physicians for teaching time.

The restriction of observations to morning work rounds conveniently answers the question of how long observations will last each day: the duration of work rounds, generally 1 to 1 1/2 hours. Still, the question remains of how many work-round sessions will be observed. In this study, the observations of work rounds will be conducted over 5 sequential days for each team being observed (Monday through Friday). The decision to focus on 5 days during 1 week is based on the premise that extended observations are necessary to obtain a detailed profile of an instructor's teaching behavior. Most studies of teaching have proceeded with a much smaller sample of teaching behavior than that called for here, but such studies are far less likely to capture an accurate picture of anyone's teaching, especially in the fluid teaching situations that occur on hospital wards. Previous findings (Weinholtz, 1981) show there is reason to believe that additional observations (beyond 6 days) yield increasingly redundant information. Thus, additional observations are ruled out as inefficient.

QUESTION 3: Will the Observations Be of Live, Videotaped, or Audiotaped Events?

Although audiotape provides a replayable record of events, its lack of a visual frame of reference makes it poorly suited for "observational" research of teaching. Hence, the decision is really one of whether or not to videotape morning work rounds. Although videotape also provides for a replayable record of events, one that can guarantee more accurate observations, videotape equipment is obtrusive and particularly ill-suited for repeated use during morning work rounds, which tend to occur virtually exclusively in the hallways and at patients' bedsides. Thus, live observations will be conducted within this study.

QUESTION 4: What Particular Instructional Behaviors Will Be Observed, and What Modus and Mechanism Will Be Used to Record the Teaching Behaviors?

Regrettably, specifying exactly which instructional behaviors will be of interest is impossible, because decisions regarding these behaviors must emerge from the preliminary descriptive study. Still, some possibilities must be given to continue this illustration. Thus, Table 8.1 addresses this issue by offering a particular observation system that derives, with minor revisions, from our research (Weinholtz et al., 1986b) on teaching by attending physicians. (For an excellent alternative approach the reader should consult Skeff et al., 1985.)

This observation system is explained in detail elsewhere (Weinholtz et al., 1986b). Here it must suffice to say that the observation system enables one to collect three types of data: (1) particular low-inference behaviors occurring during work rounds; (2) particular contexts that

TABLE 8.1 Work Round Observation System

Resident behavior	Context	Location
0. Other	0. Other	0. Other
1. Listens	1. Patient presentation or discussion	1. Conference room
2. Declares	2. Patient interview	2. Hallway
3. Positively evaluates	3. Resident examines patient	3. Bedside
4. Negatively evaluates	4. Team member examines patient	
5. Clarifying question	5. Resident prepared presentation	
6. Probing question	6. Team member prepared presentation	
7. Illustrates with prop		
8. Distributes reading		

might occur during work rounds, and (3) particular locations within which these behaviors and contexts might occur.

Briefly, the resident behaviors include nine categories: listening, declaring, verbal positive evaluations, verbal negative evaluations, clarifying questions (i.e., questions asked by the resident for his own benefit), probing questions (i.e., questions asked by the resident for pedagogical purposes), illustrating with any prop (e.g., chalkboard, x-ray viewer, EKG), distributing readings to team members, and an "other" category for all remaining behaviors (e.g., answering telephone). The "context" categories include: patient case presentations and discussions, patient interviews, patient examinations performed by the resident, patient examinations performed by other team members, prepared didactic presentations given by the resident, didactic presentation given by another team member, and an "other" category (e.g., discussion of hospital administrative policies). The location categories include the primary rounding locations (conference room, hallway, and bedside) and an "other" category (e.g., lab).

The benefit of such a system is that it has proven reliability (Weinholtz et al., 1986b), and it is likely to yield a logical set of significant correlations when the data collected using the system are matched with learning-outcomes data provided by team members (Weinholtz et al., 1986a).

As this study's "instrument" for collecting behavioral data, the observation system will be implemented using a computerized data-collection device, such as the Radio Shack Model 100™ or the Datamyte 1000™. These can be programmed to accept the system, and each contains an internal clock capable of recording amounts of time allotted to the data entries. Because they are portable and have easy program access, the computers offer tremendous advantages over the paper-and-pencil observational recording techniques that predominated just a few years ago.

QUESTION 5: What Measures Will be Adopted for Correlation with the Teaching Behaviors?

Some argue that, to be rigorous, correlational studies of teaching behaviors must correlate learner-cognitive or psychomotor skill measures with teaching behaviors. Although that notion is appealing, learner ratings of teaching effectiveness are the preferred measure here for three reasons: (1) the feasibility problems of designing cognitive or psychomotor skill tests on a large-scale study of clinical teaching behavior are overwhelming because of the many different clinical situations encountered by different ward teams; (2) reasonable correlations between learner ratings of teaching and classroom achievement tests have been demonstrated (Aleamoni, 1981); and (3) learner ratings of teaching are the measure adopted by clinical departments throughout the nation to assess teaching performance (Weinholtz et al., 1986c). Regarding this final point, because clinical departments regularly collect learner ratings of teaching performance, it makes a great deal of sense to find out what sorts of behaviors are correlated with these ratings. This argument will be even stronger in the future if standardized learner ratings begin to appear across the nation.

The specific type of learner ratings used in the study of residents' clinical teaching should be dictated by the outcomes deemed most pertinent by the investigators. Skeff et al. (1985) and my group (Weinholtz et al., 1986a) have previously adopted different types of ratings, the former involving ratings of perceived learning, the latter ratings of teacher effectiveness. For purposes of the present study, the categories in the form used by my team (Weinholtz et al., 1986a) will be adopted. The rating form (Table 8.2) will be completed by medical students, first-year residents, and any second-year residents who might be serving under a third-year resident. The form is a slightly modified subsection of a form designed by Irby (1978b) for use by the Department of Medicine at the University of Washington. The form allows for a rating of the senior residents' teaching in eight specific areas as well as an overall rating of teaching effectiveness. The specific teaching areas are: (1) knowledge of

TABLE 8.2 Resident Teaching Evaluation Form

WARD RESIDENT ________ WARD LOCATION ________ YOUR AGE ________ YOUR SEX ________ DATE ________

YOUR CLASS: Medical student ______ 3rd Year ______ 4th Year Intern ______

Directions: Please complete this form in order to evaluate the teaching of your ward resident in work rounds during the last week. Base your ratings on the ward resident's *teaching during work rounds only*.

IMPORTANT: In rating this ward resident's teaching, respond to each item carefully and thoughtfully. Avoid letting your responses to some items influence your responses to others. Keep the purpose of each section in mind as you rate the resident's teaching.

	Excellent	Very good	Good	Fair	Poor	Very poor	Not observed or applicable
1. Teaching factual knowledge, concepts and/or theories:	6	5	4	3	2	1	N
2. Teaching data collection skills (e.g., (history, lab, x-ray):	6	5	4	3	2	1	N
3. Teaching physical examination skills:	6	5	4	3	2	1	N
4. Teaching interpretation and synthesis of data:	6	5	4	3	2	1	N

5. Teaching development of patient management plans:	6	5	4	3	2	1	N
6. Teaching technical skills in diagnostic and therapeutic procedures:	6	5	4	3	2	1	N
7. Teaching interpersonal communications with patient and family:	6	5	4	3	2	1	N
8. Teaching clarity and precision in *oral* communication:	6	5	4	3	2	1	N
9. Overall, how would you rate the ward resident's teaching effectiveness:	6	5	4	3	2	1	N

10. What aspects of the resident's teaching do you feel were especially good?

11. What changes could be made to improve the resident's teaching?

concepts and theories, (2) data-collection skills, (3) physical examination skills, (4) data interpretation and synthesis, (5) patient-management plans, (6) technical skills in diagnostic and therapeutic procedures, (7) interpersonal communication with patients and families, and (8) clarity and precision in oral communications. Ratings on the items will be completed using a six-point scale ranging from "excellent" to "very poor." A "not observed" response will be included for each item. The forms will be completed at the end of each week's observations, and the respondents will be asked to focus their ratings on teaching that occurred during the work rounds conducted in the week when the observations occurred.

QUESTION 6: Will Any Additional Information Be Collected to Supplement the Behavioral and Outcomes Data?

Whenever a researcher is collecting large amounts of numerical data on behavioral phenomena, additional qualitative data must be collected to aid in the interpretation and management of the numerical data. In this study, senior residents will be interviewed briefly before the weeks they are observed, to ascertain their general teaching priorities during work rounds. Also, medical students and first-year and second-year residents will be asked to respond to two open-ended questions on their rating forms on which they are asked to describe especially strong teaching behaviors and aspects of instruction that could stand improvement. Finally, the observers will be asked to keep a brief diary in which they comment on "noteworthy" events they observed each day.

QUESTION 7: How Will the Data Collected in the Study Be Managed, Analyzed, and Interpreted?

Data management in a study of this scope demands exceptional attention to detail. The observers must enter the data daily from their portable computers onto a mainframe computer. These data must then be edited to remove error codes (e.g., one or two digits rather than three) and to discover and correct any machine malfunctions that have distorted the data (e.g., malfunctions occur occasionally in transmission from one computer to another).

The behavior data constitute one data set. The learner-ratings data constitute another. Smaller in quantity, the ratings data are much easier to manage, but equal care must be taken to assume that the data are entered properly into the computer under the code number assigned to the appropriate attending physicians. Assuming two well-groomed data sets, the raw behavioral data must be transformed into percentages of time assigned to each 3-digit, 2-digit, and single-digit codes by each senior resident. These percentages of time (per week) by senior residents can then be correlated with the ratings data. The resulting correlations can be separated into sets of correlations by different levels of team members (i.e., third-year students, fourth-year students, first-year residents, second-year residents) or sets of correlations by combined levels of team members (i.e., students, residents, or entire team).

Interpretations of findings will vary according to which sets of correlations are examined. The final challenge to the researcher in such a study is to interpret logically the correlational data in light of the qualitative data that accompany them, as well as with the existing literature in the area of interest. This interpretation is no simple feat. It requires all of the logical power necessary to interpret the qualitative data generated by descriptive studies. Some correlations that appear to have clear meaning may indeed be spurious, and vice versa. The extent to which the researchers' interpretations of correlational data are correct must eventually be determined through experimental studies.

Study 3: Experimental Evaluation of Efforts to Improve Clinical Teaching

The final study suggested here moves beyond the tentative type of confirmation provided by correlational studies to determine if teaching behaviors of interest can be manipulated through an educational intervention, and whether the resulting changes in teaching behaviors yield desired changes in associated measures (i.e., ratings of teaching effectiveness). As in the case of the correlational study (Study 2), the specific research questions to be investigated in this experimental study will depend on the research preceding it. The guidelines for Study 3 will address the seven questions dealt with in the description of Study 2, as well as an additional question regarding the educational intervention. This particular question will be addressed first.

QUESTION 1: What Sort of Educational Intervention Will Be Adopted as an Experimental Treatment?

The treatment adopted for this experimental study will be an individualized consultation similar to that adopted by Skeff (1983) and our group (Weinholtz et al., 1985a). This technique necessitates that individual clinical teachers receive feedback on their teaching derived from a preliminary round of observations. During the consultation, an educational consultant who has analyzed the resident's preliminary data will provide positive reinforcement on teaching areas where the resident has shown clear strengths, and will offer suggestions for experimentation with new teaching behaviors in areas where the resident has demonstrated relatively ineffective teaching performance. Through negotiation, the consultant will attempt to elicit a verbal contract from the resident regarding the resident's willingness to implement targeted behaviors. By necessity, those behaviors must be kept to a relatively limited number in order to prevent the task of implementing new behaviors from becoming overwhelming. A total of from two to four target behaviors seems reasonable.

The combined group of residents receiving this consultation will make up the study's treatment group. Residents participating in the study, but not receiving the consultation, will constitute the study's control group. Control group members will receive consultations after the conclusion of a second round of observations.

QUESTIONS 2 and 3: Which Residents and What Activities Will Be Observed and For How Long?

From the months of August through December, a full contingent of new second-year residents (27 residents) will be observed to obtain the preliminary data necessary for the individualized consultations. In this study, second-year residents will be chosen because they can be observed on wards where they have full ward management responsibilities, and they will have a remaining year to apply the benefits of their consultations. The contingent of residents will be randomly divided for assignment to treatment and control groups. The 27th resident will be assigned to either the treatment or control group, and will participate in the observations and consultations, but that person's data will be thrown out of the analysis to assure balanced treatment and control groups. The entire contingent of residents will again be observed during the months of January through June.

During each round of observations, work rounds will again be the only teaching activities observed. Each resident will be observed for 5 days (Monday–Friday) during each round of observations.

QUESTIONS 4, 5, and 6: Will Observations Be Live; What Instructional Behaviors Will Be Observed; and What Outcome Measures Will Be Used?

Exactly the same behavioral recording techniques as were adopted in the correlational study (Study 2) will be adopted in this experimental study. Also, exactly the same outcome measure (i.e., ratings of teaching effectiveness by team members) will be adopted.

QUESTION 7: Will Any Additional Information Be Collected to Supplement the Behavior Outcome Data?

In addition to the qualitative measures adopted in the correlational study (i.e., team member open-ended responses and observer diary comments), residents in the study will complete a brief evaluation form (Table 8.3) designed to obtain their reactions to relative benefits of the consultation process.

QUESTION 8: How Will the Data Collected in the Study Be Managed, Analyzed, and Interpreted?

Data management in the experimental study will require all of the care and attention to detail needed in the earlier correlational study. The key difference between the two will be in the type of analysis required. Rather than correlations between behaviors and ratings, the study will examine whether statistically significant differences occur between the treatment and control groups on particular criterion variables. First, the data will be analyzed to determine whether the treatment group has indeed shown changes on their selected target behaviors that are significantly greater than the changes shown on the same target behaviors by a randomly matched group of residents from the control group. Then the data will be analyzed to determine whether the learner-rating items associated with the targeted teaching behaviors have shown any significant increase in the treatment group as opposed to the control group. Finally, the overall teaching-effectiveness ratings of both groups will be compared to determine whether the treatment group's ratings have increased significantly. These results will be examined in conjunction with the resident's evaluation of the consultation process to determine the overall impact and benefits (if any) of the entire observation and consultation effort.

CONCLUSION

The combination of three studies presented here represents only one of the many possible approaches for studying clinical teaching by resi-

TABLE 8.3 Work Rounds Study—Participant Questionnaire

NAME: ____________________

Please complete this questionnaire and return via campus mail to: Donn Weinholtz, Ph.D., Office of Consultation and Research in Medical Education, 2351 Steindler Building

Circle the most appropriate answers for items 1, 2 and 3 and provide specific responses to items 4, 5 and 6.

1. I regarded my participation in this study as:	A very valuable experience 5	A valuable experience 4	A neutral experience 3	A negative experience 2	A very negative experience 1
2. The following ward residents would benefit from the type of observation and feedback that I received.	All residents 5	All new residents 4	Only volunteers 3	No residents 2	Other 1
	If "other," please explain: ____________________				
3. The Department of Internal Medicine should adopt this sort of observation and feedback procedure as standard practice for ward residents.	Yes 3	No 2	Maybe 1		
	If "maybe," please explain: ____________________				

4. Please specifically describe aspects of your participation in the study that you found valuable.

5. Please specifically describe aspects of your participation in the study that you viewed as negative or counter-productive.

6. In your opinion, how could the observations and feedback that were provided by improved?

dents. To the extent that scholarly inquiry into this type of teaching is going to develop in a rigorous, systematic, and valuable manner, it will be necessary to conduct a wide range of different descriptive, correlational, and experimental studies. Clinical teaching is an art, which can develop as a result of scientific investigation. Scientific investigation, on the other hand, is a systematic process that rests on many insightful judgments and creative designs. Much room for alternative approaches always exists within any vibrant field of investigation.

PART III

Teaching Improvement Programs for Residents: Case Examples

CHAPTER 9

Developing and Evaluating a Teaching Improvement Program for Residents

JANINE C. EDWARDS
GRACE E. KISSLING
WARREN C. PLAUCHÉ
ROBERT L. MARIER

In the spring of 1982 a program to teach residents how to teach students, patients, and peers in clinical settings was begun under the direction of the dean of the Louisiana State University (LSU) School of Medicine in New Orleans, Dr. Paul F. Larson. Dr. Larson explained his reasons in these words:

> Following a revision of the medical school curriculum, we began to focus on ways to improve the quality of the teaching efforts of the faculty. As a result of the medical students consistently mentioning the valuable, even vital, role that the house officers played as instructors, confidants and, in some instances, role models, I felt it essential to create some programs for the residents.
>
> Our resident corps, overburdened by their clinical load, often fatigued, harassed by the bureaucracy of the Charity Hospital at New Orleans and in the midst of a learning experience themselves, do not see the instruction of medical students as a primary part of their medical life. A way to

> recognize the important contribution of the residents as teachers and at the same time assist them in developing their pedagogical skills was needed. (Larson, personal communication, 1986)

The development of our program took place in two major phases: workshop development (Phase I) and videotape review with feedback (Phase II). Each phase required 2 years to implement. This case study is arranged in two portions corresponding to the different phases.

PLANNING, PHASE I

Our first planning consisted of conceptualizing the content, determining which persons to include in the program, deciding on the instructional format, laying out a timeline, and estimating the budget. In the process, we decided (1) to use a workshop format; (2) to have an educator and clinician as a team plan and teach the workshop; (3) to use as content an excellent clinical teacher's experiences and opinions combined with principles of learning theory; and (4) to require first-year house officers to attend the workshop.

The workshop method was chosen because it is familiar to medical faculty and has shown good results. Compared with other methods of educating faculty, such as individual consultation or assessment, self-instructional materials, or sabbatical leave, workshops have several advantages. The format is brief and allows active participation, which is particularly appropriate for adult learners; it isolates the participants from the work context to reduce interference with learning; and it is cost-effective because a sizable group of persons (25–35) can be taught simultaneously (Bland, 1980).

To teach the workshop we chose a team or collaborative approach because educational principles had to be applied to clinical situations. An educator and a clinical faculty member can each provide expertise in one of the two essential areas of knowledge and skill. The educator began to attend the clinician's teaching rounds, which occurred three afternoons a week. She took notes and briefly discussed the events with the clinician afterward. After several such rounds, a camera crew was brought in to videotape the rounds. Approximately 8 hours of rounds were taped during a period of 1 month.

Deciding on the content, that is, the specific clinical teaching skills to be taught, was of major importance. General principles of learning theory were selected as one type of knowledge. The monograph *Effective Clinical Teaching* (Stritter and Flair, 1980) adapted Gagné's events of instruction (1977) to clinical teaching. These principles have two advantages: (1) they have a theoretical and research base—learning theory; and (2) they are broad, general principles adaptable to a variety of settings and learners. An interactive process slowly occurred as the educator and clinician made rounds, talked together, thought about the learning principles, and viewed the videotapes.

From the beginning this program had the strong support of the dean of the medical school and the program directors involved. The dean had made it clear that residents of all specialties would be required to attend the training. Careful thought was given to selecting the level of resident. On the one hand, second-year residents have major teaching responsibilities in most programs; furthermore, by the second year, they know enough medicine to teach. On the other hand, first-year residents or interns do have some teaching responsibilities, and they may be more receptive to this type of training. The school could gain the most "mileage" from giving the teaching instruction early in the residency. Giving instruction to senior residents is too late for the institution to gain adequate return on the investment. A final consideration was that interns should be given a few months to orient themselves to their new medical responsibilities before being presented with teaching skills. Therefore, the middle of the first year of postgraduate education was chosen to initiate training in teaching skills.

DEVELOPMENT, PHASE I

The development phase involved the identification, selection, and development of objectives, content, materials, and evaluation instruments.

The following objectives were formulated for the workshop participants: (1) know the major principles of clinical teaching; (2) explain the method for teaching clinical/surgical skills; (3) give feedback to learners; and (4) have greater confidence in one's ability to teach.

To teach these objectives, four sessions were organized: a small-group discussion; a team lecture; viewing and discussing model video tapes; and role playing.

An outline of the content for the team lecture and a preliminary agenda were written. The educator studied the videotapes of teaching rounds and selected episodes illustrating particular principles of learning theory. For example, one episode illustrated the principle of transfer of learning; by relating similar cases to a difficult case at hand, the clinician tried to motivate the ward team to think comprehensively about the differential diagnosis. Another videotaped episode demonstrated the principle of directing attention—the dynamics of questioning one member of the ward team to determine what he knew about his assigned patient and how to analyze the findings systematically.

After about 3 months of planning and material development, the educator presented the plan to the clinical department heads and formally requested their support, ideas for implementation, and for outstanding senior residents to serve as an advisory committee. During the first meeting of the advisory committee, the role of these senior residents expanded in importance because they contributed excellent ideas for development of the materials and organization of the workshop. They were vitally interested and willing to give their effort to make the program a success. These residents became members of the teaching team.

The lecture outline was divided up among the team members in the first meeting. The team members discussed the educational principles to be presented, and the educator encouraged them to use their clinical experience and knowledge to develop the portion each would deliver. Background readings were provided. The complete team then began to develop cases for the role playing session. After much discussion, we decided that the team residents would play the role of students. The participants would play the role of teaching residents or observers who give feedback after the role play. The types of students to be played were standardized and written.

To practice the team lecture and role playing, two rehearsals were held before the first workshop. Each session was timed and the logistics of breaking the group into smaller groups in separate rooms were worked out.

During the first year, the educator and the department heads, residency directors, and chief residents frequently communicated about the program's purpose, its logistical arrangements, and its evaluation. This support of the clinical leaders was essential to maintaining the program.

The first time the workshop was given, it was scheduled for a full day, from 9:00 a.m. until 4:00 p.m. Participant feedback collected in writing at the conclusion indicated that the videotaped models should be shortened and the time for the entire workshop compressed. We decided to select only 2- or 3-minute videotape segments and integrate these within the team lecture. This reduced the total program time from 6 hours to 5 hours. By starting at 8:00 a.m., we fitted the workshop into half a day, which made it easier for chief residents to release their interns to attend. Coffee and lunch were provided as an added inducement for attendance.

The final workshop consisted of three sessions organized in this sequence: (1) small-group discussion; (2) team lecture with videotapes; and (3) role-playing. Table 9.1 displays the purposes, instructional methods, content, and time for each portion of the workshop.

For the first session, the small-group discussions, the stimulus questions were: "What good teaching techniques have you observed?" "What bad teaching techniques have you observed?" "What problems do you encounter in trying to teach?" Good techniques reported to the entire group usually included modeling desirable behaviors, telling students what is required on the first day of a rotation, being sensitive to the patient as a person, and discussing assigned patients and related reading with the student. Examples of bad techniques included embarrassing students in the presence of patients and causing excessive anxiety. Time to teach was always brought up as a problem. Other problems were motivating and evaluating students and interns' concern about their own level of medical knowledge.

The team of teachers capitalized on the reports from the group discussions to begin presenting new information in the second session. Whatever major points the first group included in its report were picked up and presented by team members. Interaction and discussion among the participants and teachers was thus facilitated. The team members gave personal anecdotes to make their points concrete. Differences of opinion among the participants were discussed. The videotape(s) illustrating those points was played. Then the next group was asked for its report, and so on, until all the principles had been covered. The principles of directing attention and evaluating usually had to be presented fully by the teaching team because the residents were not familiar with those ideas. Thus, we moved from group discussion slowly into a formal lecture.

References we used to develop the content for the second session included Gagné (1977) and Stritter and Flair (1980). We emphasize, however, that the experience and opinions of good clinical teachers should supersede some of the applications of educational techniques found in the medical education literature.

The major principles presented in the lecture must be applied by the residents in their everyday clinical work. To bridge the gulf between the presentation of these concepts in the lecture and the everyday world, role playing sessions were designed to provide practice and feedback. In the last session of the workshop, each participant played the role of a teaching resident or an observer of the encounter who gave feedback to the teacher. The observers were provided with a checklist of the principles of clinical teaching and were instructed to provide feedback about each of them. At the conclusion of the role playing session, all the

TABLE 9.1 Workshop on Clinical Teaching Skills

Session 1

Purposes: 1. For residents to think about teaching techniques
2. For the teachers to assess residents' awareness of teaching

Instructional method: Small-group discussions followed by reports to the entire group

Time: 30 minutes

Session 2

Purposes: 1. To provide a framework for organizing ideas about clinical teaching
2. To present educational principles that residents can apply in clinical settings
3. To model the educational principles on videotape and in the teachers' live performances

Instructional method: Team lecture with discussion illustrated with videotapes

Content: Educational principles
Communicating objectives
Communicating with patients and learners
Motivating
Directing attention
Teaching clinical/surgical procedures
Giving feedback
Evaluating

Time: 1 1/2 Hours

Session 3

Purposes: 1. To give practice with feedback
2. To allow discussion between participants and senior residents on the teaching team

Instructional method: Role playing student cases:
- A disorganized student
- An excellent student
- A student needing to learn to perform a clinical procedure

Time: Three or four 20-minute sessions

residents returned to the main room, where they wrote an evaluation of the workshop. Lunch was provided afterward.

This workshop was developed and fine-tuned during the first 2 years of our program. We have continued to give it throughout the 4 years. It serves as a general introduction that supports the residents' role as a teacher; confirms basic ideas of interaction with patients, students, and peers; and provides a framework of educational principles. Some changes are made each year because the senior residents of the teaching team change. Incorporating their suggestions keeps the experience alive. From year to year, we have noticed that those departments having a senior resident on the teaching team participate more fully and enthusiastically than the departments not having a team member. In the fall of each year, the educator meets with each team resident twice to discuss the educational principles and selected readings. One group meeting and one rehearsal are held before the first workshop is given that year. These senior residents have developed model videotapes in which they, their students, and patients serve as the actors. In all, 13 senior residents representing seven departments have been involved in the planning and teaching during the 4 years.

An educator (JE) and residency program directors (RM and WP) worked together planning every aspect of this project—holding meetings, developing materials, and winning cooperation of participants. The workshop has been given 13 times during the 4 years. Two hundred seventy house officers from 12 specialties have participated. Several clinical faculty members have also participated because they were interested in improving their own teaching.

EVALUATION

We evaluate the workshop by three methods: (1) participants' end-of-workshop evaluation form; (2) residents' self-evaluation of their teaching before and after the workshop; (3) student ratings of residents' teaching skill.

As each workshop concludes, we ask the participants to evaluate it. During the four years the workshop has been given, we have collected 195 evaluations. On these evaluations, 89% (174 participants) reported that they attained the objectives. The information presented was relevant to 93% (181). The majority of the participants also responded favorably to each of the sessions; 86% (168) thought the opening discussion was profitable; 66% (129) considered the videotapes effective, and 74% (144) thought that the role playing provided useful practice.

Self-assessment of clinical teaching skills can raise the awareness of the clinical teacher and can also be used to measure the effectiveness of instructional programs. Both purposes are served by having residents rate their clinical teaching skills before and after the workshop on the Self-Assessment Inventory for Clinical and Classroom Teaching in Medicine (Appendix I) (Irby, 1978a,b). During the 4 years (1982–1986), 105 residents rated themselves within 3 weeks prior to the workshop and again 3 to 4 months after attending the workshop. This delayed posttesting gave them time to use the educational principles. Paired *t* tests were used to analyze the pre- and postworkshop ratings. The residents rated themselves significantly higher after participating in the workshop than before it. On the eight dimensions and the summary score of the Inventory, the post–pre differences were statistically significant ($p < .01$).

Third-year students rated the teaching of the residents and faculty members on the Clinical Teaching Assessement Form (Appendix IV) at the end of each required clerkship. The student ratings of first-year residents for the 4 years (1982–1986) were analyzed statistically. We divided the student ratings into pre- and postworkshop ratings according to the dates on the rating sheets. The residents were categorized as those who had attended the workshop (Group 1) and those who had not attended (Group 2). Two group *t* tests were computed on the mean student ratings pre- and postworkshop. The students rated Group 1 significantly higher on overall teaching effectiveness ($p < .04$) afterwards than before. Group 2 was rated lower afterward than before.

The data were also analyzed by paired *t* tests (post–preworkshop mean scores) in Groups 1 and 2 separately. Although these differences were not statistically significant, the students did tend to rate the residents who attended higher on all dimensions of the inventory than those who did not attend.

In the spring of 1985, we conducted a long-term evaluation study on the effectiveness of the workshop. In addition to the results presented above, we found that at the end of their second year of residency, 94% (18 residents) of respondents to a questionnaire stated that they still considered the workshop helpful. Sixty-seven percent of those residents could recall and explain specific principles of teaching; 61% reported using principles from the course in their teaching (Edwards et al., 1986).

These results from the residents themselves and from students indicate that residents do profit from participating in a brief course on teaching skills.

PLANNING, PHASE II

As the results from the workshop evaluation began to emerge in the first year and a half, we were encouraged, but we realized that at best we were only increasing awareness and knowledge of teaching principles. Anecdotal evidence from some departments suggested that residents were teaching more frequently, but we had no objective evidence to show that residents' skill had improved. To change behaviors, more than an introductory workshop was needed. We thought that delivering instruction in clinical teaching to residents throughout the first 2 years should capitalize on the residents' developing medical knowledge and skill. Residents' teaching ability depends, to a certain extent, on medical knowledge and skill; acquiring more knowledge of the disease processes and treatments and more intellectual skill in diagnosis and performing clinical procedures naturally increases their capability and confidence as teachers (Chapters 1 and 2 of this volume). Therefore, continuing instruction about teaching during the second year seemed logical.

We decided to continue giving the workshop in the middle of the first year and to design additional support and instruction during the remainder of the first year and through the second year. The workshop presented a broad framework of principles applied to the whole spectrum of clinical teaching situations. To study the behavioral effects of the additional training, we selected one specific experience: a student presenting a patient case to a resident. Several factors made this a profitable study. The case presentation provides one of the most frequent opportunities for residents to teach students. It has fairly well-defined content and organization that is used with some variations by physicians in all specialties. Teaching students to present cases demands a range of teaching skills, including intellectual and interpersonal skills. Until recently, little explicit work had been done on teaching the case presentation (Anderson et al., 1984; Weinholtz, 1983).

In January 1984, we began to videotape residents as they taught students how to present patient cases in their normal hospital setting. This pilot work helped to focus on four questions. Can residents improve their clinical teaching skills? How do residents teach students? Which teaching skills of residents need to be improved? What methods of instruction will effect the desired improvement? The first question is primary; the other questions are instrumental in answering it.

To answer these questions, we designed a double-blind experiment. To accrue enough numbers, we combined residents from medicine, family medicine, and obstetrics and gynecology and assigned them randomly to experimental and control groups, equally matched for clinical competence. The control residents received no instruction but were required to do all of the evaluation tasks. The experimental residents received an instructional program consisting of the workshop in the middle of the first year and skill-building sessions early in their second year.

Four evaluation methods were used in a repeated measures design: (1) videotaped observations of each resident teaching a third-year student to present a patient case at the beginning of the first year, beginning of the second year, and end of the second year; (2) student rating of residents' teaching skill throughout each year; (3) resident self-rating of teaching skill at the beginning of first year, end of first year, and end of second year; and (4) questionnaire at end of workshop and end of study. We decided to collect three videotaped samples of each residents' teaching at each of the intervals to ensure adequate reliability. The total number of videotapes to be made by each experimental and control resident, therefore, was nine.

DEVELOPMENT AND IMPLEMENTATION, PHASE II

For the first year of the study (1984–1985), the baseline videotapes had to be made before the experimental residents attended the workshop. Because noise and crowded conditions in the hospitals had made videotaping there impractical, a standardized setting of chairs and chalkboard was arranged in the office building adjoining the hospital. All videotapes for the 2-year study were made in this setting. Collecting the videotapes proved to be more difficult than we had anticipated and required 4 months instead of 2 months. The residents found it difficult not only to find the time to do this task, but also to persuade students to accommodate them. However, the work was eventually completed as planned. The workshops were given in the middle of the year; the experimental residents from the study as well as residents from all other specialties attended.

Development of the instruction and evaluation of the new program proceeded simultaneously; this ensured a close match between what would be taught and evaluated. In the spring of 1985, three research assistants, who were psychology graduate students from a local university, began to work with us. The full team consisted of the educator, both the medicine and obstetrics and gynecology residency directors, a family medicine faculty member, and the graduate students. We began to study the pilot videotapes intensely and to refine the first-draft evaluation instruments. The ideas that shaped the evaluation instruments were translated into instructional materials and live teaching activities. We tried out a series of three pilot skill-building sessions for second-year residents; these seemed to be moderately successful. Slowly the team developed specific descriptions of the range of teaching behaviors observed on the first- and second-year residents' videotapes and on the model videotapes made by senior residents and faculty.

In September 1985, we were ready to launch the series of three small-group skill-building sessions for the experimental residents. Our plan was to present an overview of the strategy we had developed to teach case presentations, and then to teach each phase of the strategy in detail in two sessions spaced 1 month apart. In between each session the experimental residents would make one videotape and review it independently. The control residents would also make the videotapes but would receive no review or instruction. The teaching team consisted of the educator, a clinician, and two senior residents. For the first session, we had produced a model videotape, and colored slides and charts illustrating the strategy, rehearsed the session, and communicated with everyone concerned. We had prepared well, but we had inklings of difficulty because the second-year residents were becoming resistant.

We expected a maximum of 11 residents; 5 showed up. All groused about having to make videotapes and became openly hostile when we tried to interact with them about teaching techniques. They complained that no one had given them feedback about the videotapes they had made the first year. One seemed to voice the feelings of the majority when he said, "My residency director has never given me feedback about these tapes. I'm not getting anything out of this." Another one said, "This is just another bureaucratic thing, someone sitting in an office dreaming up more paperwork for us to do, answerin' questionnaires, comin' to teaching conferences. None of us want to do this." Our explanations about the study had little positive effect on the residents' negative attitude.

After that session, we determined to explain the purpose and design of the study more fully to the residents. We decided to acknowledge that half of the residents were control subjects. It also seemed obvious that we should use the actual videotapes the residents had made instead of model videotapes, as we had planned. We had to offer some incentive to all of them to continue with the study, the difficulty of making the videotapes had to be eased, and the instruction for the experimental group had to be meaningful. Negotiations took several weeks. The chairman and the residency directors of the three departments did not back down. They continued to support the program. Compromises were reached so that the experimental study could continue.

In November we began again with a plan that succeeded over the next 5 months. Open communication about the purposes and operation of the study was essential. The residency director and the educator met with the second-year residents in each program to explain the study and ask for their cooperation. We acknowledged that we had tried to conduct the study as a double-blind experiment and that had not worked. We offered small financial stipends as an incentive to every resident for completing each phase of the study. Coming forward openly and admitting our mistakes changed the residents' negative attitude. They ventilated their frustrations and made suggestions about how to proceed. We implemented many of these.

We made two key changes in our instructional plan. Instead of grouping residents across specialties (medicine, family medicine, and obstetrics and gynecology) for instruction, the residency director of each program and the educator worked with each specialty separately. We decided to give the experimental residents what they asked for—feedback on the videotapes they had made, not generalized model videotapes. Feedback sessions were scheduled with groups of two, three, or four residents. Each session lasted about an hour.

In the first round of sessions, we presented the charts illustrating the teaching strategy. Then we played the most recent tape of each resident or portions of it. The residency director gave the first feedback and engaged the individual resident in discussion. The educator gave additional feedback and usually opened the discussion to the entire group. In the second round of sessions, we praised the improvement we noted in comparison with the previous performance, reviewed the teaching strategy, noted specific points needing further work, and discussed teaching problems individual residents were encountering with their teams. We tried to assist the residents in transferring the teaching principles from the context of a case presentation to their everyday teaching situations. No resident objected to having other residents see his tapes. The residency director's feedback seemed most important to each person. Some of the problems discussed were motivating students to learn, finding time to teach as well as to take care of patients, managing a ward team, educating patients, and requiring patient-centered reading of students. Giving feedback in small groups enabled each resident to see a range of teaching behaviors and to discuss a range of techniques, and it also controlled the total amount of time required. These critique sessions satisfied the experimental residents. The experimental residents made two videotapes and participated in two peer-review sessions. The controls simply made two videotapes during this same period.

We devised a strategy for teaching presentations that we used in our skill-building sessions (Figure 9.1). For purposes of analysis, a case presentation can be divided into three phases. Phase I of the case presentation can be termed Organizing and Reporting Patient Information. A

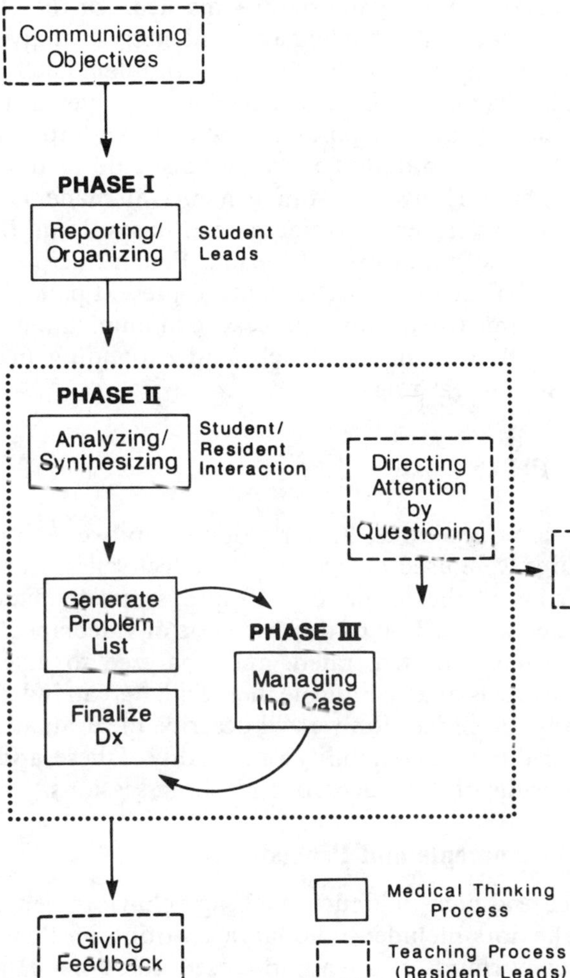

FIGURE 9.1 Teaching skills for three phases of a case presentation.

long and short form are used, depending on the service. Generally, the long form is used on medicine-oriented services and the short form on surgically oriented services. In our study, internal medicine and family medicine belonged to the first group and obstetrics and gynecology belonged to the second group. The long form includes the chief complaint, history of the present illness, medical history, social history, family history, medication, allergies, review of systems, physical examination findings, and laboratory data. The short form includes only the chief complaint, pertinent positive history, and physical findings.

Phase II is Analyzing and Synthesizing—the heart of the clinical reasoning process. Together the resident and student try to analyze and synthesize the patient information to generate a problem list and formulate a differential diagnosis. They need to relate the patient information to pathophysiology and to possible etiologies. A problem list should be generated and a differential diagnosis should be discussed for each problem. Phase III involves Management—all matters regarding further evaluation (work-up) and treatment. Phases II and III give the resident the greatest opportunity to teach. Four principles from learning theory can be used to assist students to present patient cases and engage in the clinical reasoning process: communicating objectives, directing attention, giving feedback, and expanding the case (teaching for transfer of learning).

EVALUATION, PHASE II

The primary research question is, "Can residents improve their teaching?" Four measures were used to evaluate the effectiveness of the instruction. The results of the residents' self-ratings and the students' ratings are presented above. Two of the three sets of videotapes in the experiment have been collected, rated, and analyzed to date. The results from these two sets of data indicate that residents can indeed improve their teaching. In this section we will describe the evaluation instruments and procedures, the reliability and validity of these, and indicate preliminary results of the videotaped teaching sessions.

The Evaluation Instruments and Procedures

Both low-inference and high-inference teaching behaviors were rated. Low-inference behaviors included note taking, writing on the chalkboard, and frequency counts of open and closed questions. High-inference behaviors included communicating objectives, directing attention during the students' initial presentations, formulating the differential diagnosis, deciding and evaluating treatment, expanding the case, optimizing the quality of learning climate, giving feedback, and acknowledging limitations. These high-inference behaviors were rated on a scale of 1 (low) to 6 (high). Each point on the scale was defined by verbal anchors describing behaviors observed on a wide range of teaching videotapes. The student's performance was rated as average, above average, or below average. The final rating given for each tape was a holistic judgment of the quality of teaching performance; it was not an average of previous ratings.

Two raters, both blind to experimental and control groups memberships, rated each videotape independently. Most of the tapes were 15 to 20 minutes long. The raters evaluated the first 15 minutes of every tape. Although some tapes necessitated five viewings to be rated completely, the raters were able to complete their ratings for most tapes after three viewings. The student performance was one of the first things rated because the teaching process is interactive. The teacher must adapt his techniques to the ability and performance of the learner. Only after making a judgment about the student's performance could the raters evaluate the teacher's skill in directing attention to the diagnosis and treatment, for example.

Validity Study

In a study of this type, the question naturally arises, "Could persons unfamiliar with medical content validly rate the teaching skills of persons engaged in a medical dialogue?" In developing the instruments and procedures, the educator and psychology graduate students (i.e., the raters) had worked with four physicians. However, as an additional check, a formal validity study was conducted. Comparisons were made between ratings by the clinician (WP), the educator (JE), and the two raters.

Seven videotapes were selected for rating: two first-year controls, two first-year experimentals, one second-year control, and two second-year experimentals. Two residents were from family medicine; one from obstetrics and gynecology; and four from medicine.

On the 11 scales of the seven tapes, 385 possibilities for agreement/disagreement existed (11 scales x 5 comparisons x 7 tapes). "Agreement" was judged to occur when both raters evaluated the tape on the same side of the scale (i.e., positive or negative). Agreement was obtained on 358 pairs (93%) of ratings. On the three teaching-skill scales mentioned above (differential diagnosis, expanding the case, and managing the case), agreement was obtained on 85 out of 105 possible pairs of ratings (81%).

The second criterion for validity was for ratings to be no more than one point apart. A total of 308 ratings were made (4 raters x 7 tapes x 11 scales). Only 13 out of 308 ratings (4%) were actually more than one point apart. Thus, 96% of the ratings met this criterion.

On average, both raters agreed with the physician and educator in their scoring of the seven tapes (paired *t* tests). The only significant disagreement occurred between the educator and physician. The educator on average rated the residents higher on expanding the case than did the physician. These results indicate substantial agreement between a physician and nonphysicians in the rating of teaching skills.

Reliability

Reliability studies were done at three times; the results of the third study are reported here. Two questions were addressed: "How consistent is each rater?" "What is the interrater reliability?" Each rater was consistent in her ratings. This consistency was checked by having each rater periodically rate tapes a second time. Paired *t* tests between first and second ratings were computed for each scale. Potential biases by specialty and by treatment group (experimental or control) were examined by analysis of variance. No significant biases were found.

Interrater reliability was confirmed by computing Pearson product-moment correlations and paired *t* tests on the scores given by the two raters on the same resident. On the 14 scales, the correlations ranged from .65 to 1.00, with the exception of directing attention during the student's presentation, which had a correlation of .26. All correlations were statistically significant at or beyond the 0.001 level. The correlation for the summary rating was .73.

The evaluation instruments and procedures in this study showed adequate validity and reliability.

Comparison of the Experimental and Control Videotapes

Preliminary analyses of two thirds of the total number of videotapes in the experiment have been completed. The two raters' scores for each scale for each tape were averaged to obtain an assessment of the resident's teaching ability. Two sample *t* tests were computed between the experimental and control groups before instruction, and again during the instruction in the second year. Two-way analysis of variance (treatment group × time) was also computed.

The paired *t* tests revealed that during the second year the experimental residents had improved their teaching skills on every one of the scales, and they scored higher than the control residents on eight of the nine scales. In contrast, the control residents' skills had remained the same or declined slightly during the year and a half. On four of the five scales (communicating objectives, directing the student's presentation, expanding the case, learning climate, and overall) the difference between experimental and control residents was statistically significant at the 0.05 level.

These preliminary results seem to indicate that residents can improve their teaching skills.

CONCLUSION

Our experiences in bringing about this improvement demonstrate that the active support of the clinical leaders—departments heads, residency directors, and chief residents—is critical in maintaining a program to teach residents how to teach. If the residency directors had not been involved in the instruction, the residents would not have accepted the program.

A team composed of an educator, residency directors, and chief residents can function effectively. Giving the chief residents some intensive instruction each year is a repetitive task, but it is worthwhile. They are the closest role models for resident teachers, they handle the logistics of scheduling, and they contribute new vitality to the program each year.

We used a combination of instructional methods: an introductory workshop during the middle of the first year and peer review with feedback of residents' own videotapes during the middle of the second year. The workshop provides awareness of the teaching role and a framework of educational principles. The videotape reviews hone the skills of teaching.

The total instructional time required was 8 hours—5 hours for the workshop, 1 hour for making videotapes, and 2 hours for peer review of the tapes. In our experiment, additional time was required for evaluation work, but this is not part of the instructional program. Eight hours of instruction is feasible to implement, especially when one considers the benefit to the residents (see Chapter 1).

We are convinced that the timing of the instruction is important. We began the instruction in December of the first year and concluded it in March of the second year. Residents are on a steep learning vector in the first and second years of residency. Instruction in teaching skill should be timed to capitalize on this vector (Chapter 2, p. 20).

We have also learned some important things about conducting evaluation research of resident teaching. Heavy demands for evaluation will interact negatively with an instructional program. A balance between instruction and evaluation has to be maintained. When residents are subjects in a study, open communication with them about their roles is essential. For our control residents, feedback was more desirable than a stipend. Of course, the stipend was not rejected, but many would have preferred to receive feedback about their teaching. We conclude that residents do recognize their teaching role and want to improve themselves as teachers.

Establishing teaching-skills programs as an integral part of residency programs generally will depend on development of materials that are relevant to clinicians, as well as approaches that are time-effective, fit into the daily clinical routines, and can be maintained by the clinical leaders without the presence of an educator. We have shown that residents' teaching skills can be improved. Now the task is to determine how best to integrate instruction about teaching into residency-program routines.

CHAPTER 10

The Children's Hospital Experience

LARRIE W. GREENBERG
LESLIE S. JEWETT
RHONDA M. GOLDBERG

> Education does not mean teaching people to know what they do not know; it means teaching them to behave as they do not behave.
>
> —John Ruskin

As fourth-year medical students anxiously anticipate entering their residencies, another developmental step in their lifelong training, few in their undergraduate curricula will have had the opportunity to study and learn some of the essential skills they will use as residents and throughout their professional careers. One skill is effectiveness in teaching.

Teaching is an important responsibility residents must assume during their training. Residents spend about 20% to 25% of their time teaching parents, patients, and students (Brown, 1970). Yet, most residents do not have formal training in teaching, learning how to teach by observing clinicians and more senior residents who are role models in the clinical setting and who teach in a traditional, authoritarian way (Cantrell, 1973).

Helping residents acquire effective teaching skills during their residency is now gaining emphasis. The Accreditation Council for Graduate Medical Education (ACGME) in its *Directory of Residency Training Programs* states that programs should assist residents in acquiring skills in teaching and evaluating those for whom they are responsible (American Medical Association, 1986). The guidelines also state that "clinical departments are expected to organize formal teaching sessions tailored to meet the special requirements of their programs." The Association of American Medical Colleges also recognizes the importance of teaching skills for physicians. In its report on the General Professional Education of the Physician (GPEP), the AAMC advocates the need for more effective teachers who have skills that promote problem-solving and self- directed learning (Association of American Medical Colleges, 1984).

Here we describe the development and implementation of a teaching skills training program for residents based on our experiences.

DEVELOPMENT OF THE CHILDREN'S HOSPITAL NATIONAL MEDICAL CENTER (CHNMC) TEACHING PROGRAM

The idea for developing a residency teaching skills training program at CHNMC began in 1978, at which time we perceived that residents needed to be more effective teachers. A review of the literature revealed a flurry of activity in teaching skills at the faculty level, but minimal involvement with residents. We developed a grant proposal and submitted it to the National Fund for Medical Education. In July 1979, soon after the proposal was accepted, our teaching skills training program began. The overall project goal was to improve the quality of resident teaching delivered to medical students by training residents to teach more effectively (Jewett et al., 1982b).

Participants

Residents at all three levels of training were selected to participate in the program. Each training level of residents was randomly divided into experimental and control groups. We were aware that interns (PGY-1s) are traditionally preoccupied with cognitive issues such as how to resuscitate patients, manage their time effectively, write orders independently, and establish credibility with the group they are expected to teach, that is, the medical students. Learning teaching skills and techniques is certainly not considered top priority within this context. Some authorities, however, estimate that interns teach for about

10% of their working day (Alpert, 1973); however, that percentage may be decidedly underestimated, because interns spend time with medical students in dyads, group settings, and unplanned informal hallway encounters, as well as on the telephone (Greenberg and Jewett, 1983). Offering a teaching program early in a resident's training enables the trainee to build on these skills throughout his 3 or more years of apprenticeship. Training program directors who are forced by limited resources to start such a teaching program at one level only should be aware that including more experienced residents who have acquired a sizable knowledge base and who have already adapted to the hospital routine would be optimal. Experienced trainees have fewer pressures, are closer to completion of training, and are likely to be more concerned about specific skills—including those pertaining to teaching—that they will need for their careers.

To improve the quality of their teaching, residents participated in a variety of educational activities before and after the intervention in this study design—two workshops on clinical teaching skills and two sessions of feedback on their teachings. These activities included the following: (1) completion of a questionnaire both before the implementation of a clinical teaching program and after the experimental group participated in the workshops; (2) completion of instruments focusing on learning and teaching preferences and interpersonal styles that we hypothesized would impact on or correlate with teaching, namely, the FIRO-B (Fundamental Interpersonal Relationships Orientation Behavior) (Shutz, 1966), the LPI (Learning Preference Inventory of Rezler) (Rezler and French, 1975), and the TMPs (Teaching Management Problems) (Jewett et al., 1982a); and (3) critique of five videotaped, nonrehearsed teaching sessions in the clinics and on the wards.

The questionnaire focused on residents' perceptions of teaching and learning in undergraduate and graduate training. The content was based on our own experience, a literature review, and a questionnaire developed by Meleca and Schimpfhauser (1976). The objectives were to assess the residents' perceptions of teaching as a responsibility; their role as teachers; teaching methods, styles, and skills; and means for improving clinical teaching (Greenberg et al., 1984). The questionnaire was also designed to determine whether the residents' confidence as teachers related to their perceptions toward specific aspects of teaching and learning.

Program Evaluation

One of the most difficult and yet important aspects of educational research is a well-planned evaluation that reflects the program's goals and objectives. Ideally an evaluation should monitor the ongoing program, be proactive to problems, and assess the impact of the workshop on resident teaching skills. Two important aspects to consider in designing an evaluation are the methods of measurement and the resources.

In determining an evaluation method, consideration must be given to the dramatic changes occurring in the health care industry, specifically in that cost is the major determinant of beginning or continuing any activity. The evaluation must be designed to measure the benefits the teaching skills program will bring to the institution and to those directly involved in the program: the residency training program director, the chief residents, the residents, and the administration.

Once the benefits of the program have been stipulated, it is important to specify which available evaluation methods will be used for measuring program objectives. Other case studies within this book are good resources for evaluation methodology. Communicating with directors who have administered previous teaching skills programs can also be helpful. We recommend selecting subjective and objective methods, if possible, and those that require minimal time to administer and analyze in deriving the information needed.

Resources

Adequate evaluation requires resources. Evaluation must be a built-in cost to the teaching skills program. The type of evaluation depends on the financial support for personnel in each program. If financial support is not available, using personnel such as administrative staff already present within a department to monitor and collect data is cost-effective. In addition, use of graduate students is also recommended, inasmuch as some of them may be seeking experience or places in which to do course projects.

PROGRAM IMPLEMENTATION

Coordination of the activities to implement the proposed plan is a key to the program's success. An organizational process must be developed that ensures the plan will be carried out exactly as specified. Important features of the implementation are as follows.

Staff

The tasks that need to be done before, during, and at the completion of the program must be specified and analyzed, and the amount of time each will take determined. The task analysis will depend on your specific program's scope. Next, decide which responsibilities will be assumed by different staff members and whether financial support is available to hire other staff, such as a consultant to be the instructor, a research assistant, or project coordinator if the program warrants.

Of great value to the success of implementing the program is a project coordinator, in managing and delegating the specific tasks and in monitoring ongoing activities. The administrative time commitment may be minimal or extensive, depending on the amount of available support staff. We recommend that part-time administrative support be made available for the scheduling and distribution of reminders for meetings and workshops. If financial support is limited, graduate students from a local university should be considered. Some are interested in gaining experience or use programs such as these as a practicum requirement, even if they receive no pay. Other funding to consider should include grants awarded from outside or within the institution, or a line-item commitment in the departmental budget.

At CHNMC, ours was a research project and required two part-time research assistants to do the actual research, a program coordinator (20% time), a secretary (20% time), the consultant to provide the instruction, and the project director and two co-directors. This project had outside funding, and most of the time spent by the staff was directed toward the research part of this project. The staffing size should not discourage anyone who wants to develop a teaching skills program.

Orientation

Important to the implementation of a new program is a proper orientation for those who will participate in it. At CHNMC, the orientation provided an opportunity for the residents to become familiar with the overall goals and objectives of the teaching skills program, to learn how it would benefit them, to discuss their questions and concerns, and to take part in the scheduling. The residency training program director (RTPD) and/or the chief residents should clearly explain the goals and objectives of the program and the other specific program information at the orientation, with others who are directly involved also in attendance to answer specific questions.

Residents attended either of two orientations, each given at an early morning breakfast at the beginning of the study. Minimizing inconvenience to the residents is crucial to the success of any such program. Residents need sufficient lead time to schedule nonpatient activities. For this reason, at the orientation they were given a schedule of the workshops for the year. About 1 week after the orientation, residents in the experimental group were given the choice of times that they could select to participate in the workshops. Each workshop was offered at three different times during a 2-day period. This scheduling process was repeated with the control group residents in the spring of 1980, when the study was completed.

The Ongoing Program

Once the program begins, the RTPD, administration, and chief residents should be kept informed of the program's progress. Communication should underscore the positive effects of the training (unless it is conducted as research) and be sufficiently open to identify and solve problems as they arise. Residents participating in the program should have an opportunity while it is ongoing to express their satisfactions and dissatisfactions and be aware that the program is responsive to their needs.

INTERVENTION

The intervention used in this study comprised two half-day workshops and two 1-hour instructional sessions consisting of group and individual consultations on teaching. Twenty-seven residents in the experimental group participated in these exercises in November 1979 and April 1980, whereas the control group received no instruction until after the completion of the study. The focus of the workshops was to help residents develop problem-based teaching techniques and for them to encourage the active participation of students and peers in the learning process, with the purpose of developing the learner's clinical problem-solving skills. The workshops were conducted by a recognized authority on faculty development and teaching. This person also provided consultation on program development, implementation, and evaluation strategies. We were of the opinion that contracting with an outside consultant might be more conducive for residents to be open in learning new teaching skills and in modifying others.

The first 3-hour workshop was presented after we were able to collect baseline data on all residents, using the questionnaire, instruments, and videotapes as outlined above. One of the first tasks in the workshop was for residents to recall the most effective teacher with whom they interacted and to describe the characteristics that made that teacher unique. The consultant then presented the residents with a standardized form that they were to use as an evaluation tool to rate teaching effectiveness of two videotaped teaching situations. The tapes illustrated two styles of teaching: (1) traditional didactic instruction, in which the teacher provides information and the student is a passive learner and (2) the student-oriented or Socratic approach, in which the instructor encourages and assists the student to learn by synthesizing collected data and using the problem-solving method. With this evaluation form, the residents were able to differentiate between the two teaching methods and understand the importance of active learning.

The initial 1-hour optional session was offered 1 to 2 months after the first workshop. The focus of the session, which was informal and during lunch, was to discuss strategies learned in the first workshop and applications of the FIRO-B, the LPI, and the TMP instruments to improve teaching and learning in the clinical setting. The FIRO-B, first developed for industry as a means to determine a person's interpersonal characteristics and how well they fit in with the job environment, has a significant correlation with how one chooses to teach (Jewett et al., 1982b). The FIRO-B is based on the assumption that all human interaction may be divided into three categories; (1) inclusion, (2) control, and (3) affection. The instrument has two dimensions: interpersonal areas and direction of one's behavior, which is what one expresses to and wants from others. A high score means a preference and need for interaction with others, whereas a low score suggests the desire to limit contact with people. Using this instrument with resident physicians, we hypothesized that the resident's FIRO-B profile and interest would correlate significantly with his effectiveness in teaching.

The LPI originally was used with other health care professionals and more recently with physicians (Rezler and French, 1975). This instrument enables a person to examine how he prefers to learn. It also enables residents to understand that physicians have different learning styles and that these can have a positive or negative impact on teaching. Categories making up the Rezler LPI include abstract, concrete, teacher-structured, student-structured, interpersonal, and independent learning.

The TMPs, similar in format to patient management problems (PMPs) as used by the National Board of Medical Examiners, were developed by us to assess a resident's pencil-and-paper approach to various teaching situations. Ten problems simulating the clinical setting were presented during the year. An example of a TMP included a senior pediatric resident deciding how much independence to give a rotating family practice resident who had no pediatric experience after medical school with regard to patient care and decision-making. The scoring system is based on whether the teacher or learner assumes responsibility for each action taken in the problem.

The second 1-hour optional session took place after the final workshop. Residents were offered another opportunity with the use of their videotapes to assess their teaching by means of the problem-based approach. Discussion focused on reviewing the strengths and strategies for further refinement of teaching skills that enhance problem-solving and student interaction.

RESULTS

Evaluation methods used in the CHNMC program included a pretest-posttest control design to study the impact of the workshops on resident teaching behavior. The questionnaire that the residents completed pre- and postworkshop showed that those residents in the experimental group expressed more self-confidence in their teaching (Greenberg et al., 1984). Residents who reported confidence in their teaching consider this responsibility a priority and enjoyed working with students. This expressed confidence also correlated significantly with their style and management of teaching, and with their approach to teaching in an organized and logical manner. In addition to their increased self-confidence after the workshop intervention, peers, students, and faculty consistently rated the teaching of residents who had received instruction higher than that for residents who had had no instruction.

The FIRO-B revealed some interesting differences between the residents in the experimental and control groups. Residents with the most confidence in, and positive evaluations and feedback about, their teaching were found to have (1) moderate (46%) or high (25%) needs to exercise authority over others, (2) moderate needs for control or authority from others (71%), and (3) high needs to be liked and to gain approval from others (54%) (Jewett et al., 1983). These residents differed significantly from peers who had little confidence in, and lower evaluations and less positive feedback about, their teaching. This group had (1) minimal need to express authority over others (71%), (2) high (24%) or low needs (45%) for authority from others, and (3) moderate or low needs for approval or to be liked by others (66%).

Residents with strong desires for contact with people and close relationships preferred learning activities that involved others ($r = +.46$, $p < .0007$). Residents who prefer to be alone and have business-like relationships were more likely to prefer independent learning, such as reading ($r = -.33$, $p < .01$), self-directed learning activities ($r = -.44$, $p < .001$), and abstract learning ($r = -.30$, $p < .03$). As has been shown in other studies on physicians, most residents (67%) prefer concrete learning (Jewett et al., 1983).

Another important evaluation method was to create an interaction analysis for the teaching–learning situation based on the instrument developed by the National Board of Medical Examiners (NBME) for the doctor–patient interaction (Flanders, 1974). Each resident participated in five videotaped, unrehearsed teaching encounters throughout the year. We hypothesized that these sessions could be objectively rated using the modified instrument described above. Categories rated including giving commands or directions; responding with questions; initiating topics or making statements; being silent or showing uncertainty. Nonphysicians were trained to record the resident's behavior every 3 seconds to assess teaching behaviors and patterns. Although these data have not been formally published and are in the data-entry stage, this method is an objective way to evaluate teaching.

PROBLEMS

If the departmental chairperson and the RTPD do not actively support the program, the residents will be aware of that lack of leadership from those persons and the program will fail. It is advisable to delegate some responsibility to either or both of these persons as evidence that the program has support and encouragement from the administration itself.

Realistically, residents are unlikely to receive such a program with unabashed enthusiasm for several reasons: (1) They are not generally aware that there is a body of knowledge regarding teaching and learning and that skills that have been traditionally learned "on the job" can be taught from the theoretical and clinical perspectives. (2) This issue will have a lower priority because the residents' curriculum is already cramped. (3) Most residents, because they have not done a self-assessment on their own teaching skills, have not established the need to improve. (4) Residents who receive positive feedback from students on their teaching perceive themselves as "good" teachers. (5) Few faculty members who are role models have participated in such training.

Other potential problems previously mentioned include cost of the program, a workable evaluation methodology, and collection and analysis of the data to provide the participants with feedback.

Finally, expectations of the outcome of such a program should be realistic. Only a few residents are likely to actually apply newly learned skills to the clinical setting, but this should not be a deterrent to starting the program. In any field change is difficult and requires a self-assessment of the level at which one is functioning, an appreciation of the level at which one ought to be performing, and motivation on how to change to the better level. Those residents who change their teaching behaviors by promoting more problem- solving and effective learning in students and peers will be better role models. Through this process, change will take place and teaching will be more effective.

PROGRAM CONTINUATION AND DISSEMINATION

The final step in establishing an effective program is ensuring that the program continues once it is completed. Many of the strategies have already been discussed, such as evaluation and financial and administrative support. This stage is the control process to determine whether the objectives and benefits set in the planning and development steps are being met. When objectives are not met, ways must be developed to change the program to meet them.

Program Continuation

After the final teaching skills program is evaluated, planning must resume again, based on the evaluation. A concise report outlining the program and its important outcomes should be used to initiate planning with the RTPD, the present and the future chief residents, and the administration. A pitfall to avoid is taking too long to develop the final program report. Timeliness and responsiveness in evaluation are key factors in program continuation.

The planning process must proceed again and recycle. If the program has positive findings, these can be used not only as a selling point on program continuation but also as support for financial commitments from the institution.

Dissemination

If the program is successful, residents in other departments may want to participate in a teaching skills program. The institution may also want to consider teaching skills training as a medical school agenda issue through the Graduate Education Committee (GEC). A commitment by the medical school rather than at a departmental level could assist departments with expenses and possibly personnel.

OUTGROWTHS OF THE CHNMC

Several new programs have been developed a teaching skills program and research conducte vths from the have been directed to two groups: faculty and stu MC. These

Curricula for faculty workshops have been devel the special needs of full-time and voluntary faculty in t cusing on ambulatory units. Education in the inpatient setting usu tient and the group setting with a specific schedule (i.e., attendir curs in rounds, work rounds), whereas teaching in the ambulatory d ching involves the student, resident, and teacher in a one-to-one s ment throughout the day as they care for patients. Curricula for tion workshops are based on participant needs and responsibilities i se the educational system, although the same educational principles are used as are applicable to our residency program. With voluntary faculty members who teach in their offices or in community hospitals, practical management may be stressed. The emphasis may differ for full-time faculty who teach in a medical school or affiliated hospital.

A 2-week, fourth-year medical student elective has also been offered in teaching. One or two students participate at one time during the elective and read selected literature on problem-based, interactive learning, adult learning, teaching and learning skills, and other related topics. Students then discuss these issues in a seminar with one of us. They also observe and evaluate teaching in different settings (inpatient, critical care units, ambulatory department) and formats (grand rounds, teaching rounds, attending rounds) within the hospital, applying principles of reading and the seminars to these situations. Then, they have an opportunity to apply what they have learned from the elective by leading a videotaped teaching session with third-year students and receiving feedback.

For senior medical students after match day, a one-half day workshop is offered to acquaint them with some of the teaching skills they will use as PGY-1s. The workshop includes microteaching sessions in which students are able to apply principles in a simulated teaching session.

SUMMARY

The teaching skills training program for residents is an effective technique that can improve their instruction with relatively little time (about 8 ho al participation) and expense. To be successful, programs e one developed at Children's Hospital must be based on nal and residents' needs. Effective planning, program de nt, evaluation, implementation, and continuation strategi e essential elements of an effective teaching skills program fo ents.

CHAPTER 11

Teaching Surgery Residents to Teach

C. BENJAMIN MELECA
JAMES A. PEARSOL

Dave*, a second-year resident in general surgery, is really pressed today. He assisted Dr. Mara in a long operation yesterday, and he is behind on his own patient write-ups. Sheila is a third-year clerk beginning her second week in general surgery. She is curious about the oncological nutritionist's dietary recommendations for Mrs. Caale. She asks Dave, "Why are you actually restricting Mrs. Caale's diet?"

Dave faced a decision choice. Teaching in surgery by nature and design seems a random occurrence, but it is a form of teaching that ideally develops from and through the real experiences of surgical patients. Dave is a good teacher. He realized that some of the best lessons learned in surgery come through understanding patients' problems and therapeutic management. Although strapped for time, Dave spent 5 more minutes with Sheila to explain the nutritional component of Mrs. Caale's treatment plan.

Dave asked, "Sheila, what are you wondering?" Sheila responded, "It seems to me that with her loss of weight, we should be feeding her more, not less." Dave went on to explain that there was some research evidence suggesting that increased caloric intake actually causes a tumor to grow. "In

*Note: all names used are fictitious.

Mrs. Caale's case it is important to permit a minor weight loss to reduce the risk of cancer spread."

This brief example introduces one of the key concepts underlying our approach to teaching residents to teach—to recognize and take advantage of one's opportunity and responsibility to teach at the teachable moment. Dave capitalized on Sheila's request and responded, first by seeking more information about the nature of her request, then by explaining the purpose of Mrs. Caale's nutrition plan.

At the Ohio State University College of Medicine, residents are largely responsible for the teaching of third- and fourth-year medical students and fellow house officers. Second only to patient care and their own clinical training, house staff spend a great amount of time in teaching or teaching-related activities. An early survey of house staff teaching responsibilities at Ohio State revealed three unsurprising pieces of information. First, 50% to 75% of information received by medical students during their clerkship experiences came from the house staff. Second, few residents had had any formal preparation for teaching. Third, although residents considered teaching of medical students an important responsibility to be shared by faculty and attending physicians, such teaching was definitely not a priority among a list of residents' responsibilities. Teaching was preceded by their own continuing medical education and training and by patient care. Today we conclude that our experiences at Ohio State operate under the same conditions as existed previously.

The program we describe represents our attempt to develop resident teachers-in-training.[1] We knew we faced limited opportunity for teaching residents to teach (because of the demands on their time). We also knew that residents teach in varied environments. Our approach was to design a seminar that introduced a wide range of instructional strategies and productive teaching behaviors, all within the constraint of limited access and resources.

PLANNING AND DEVELOPMENT OF THE SEMINAR

Getting the surgical residents' teaching skills program off the ground necessitated that different offices and departments work together to

1. It is important to note that the teaching skills "program" evolved into a 1-day, 8-hour seminar. It is doubtful that such an event qualifies as a resident training program in teaching skills. However, the extensive planning process (described here) for the 1-day seminar laid the groundwork for periodic educationl skills sessions above and beyond an annual teaching skills seminar. Enhancements to the 1-day seminar are described in greater detail in our conclusions and recommendations. Throughout this chapter we use the words "program" and "seminar" interchangeably.

satisfy a perceived need. The Division of Research and Evaluation in Medical Education (DREME), an academic service unit within the dean's office in the College of Medicine, is staffed by seven professional educators having expertise in curriculum and instruction, in educational research and evaluation, and in testing and measurement. We worked with the Department of Surgery Undergraduate Education Committee to plan the seminar. The way the planning started is an example of matchmaking by word-of-mouth.

Getting Started

Dr. Simpson, chair of the College of Medicine's Executive Curriculum Committee, is a faculty member of the Department of Surgery. At a September Executive Curriculum Committee meeting, he listened to another faculty member describing a house staff teaching skills seminar conducted by the staff of DREME for the Department of Medicine. Dr. Simpson was eager to have a similar program for surgical house staff. He arranged for us to meet with the chair of the Department of Surgery and the chair of the Department's Undergraduate Education Committee. At that meeting we agreed to proceed with planning of a house staff teaching skills program for all surgical house staff.

A series of meetings followed to define what such a teaching skills program might entail. For Dr. Briggs, the chair of the Undergraduate Education Committee, planning a program of teaching skills for residents was a familiar assignment. In 1974 a pilot clinical teaching program was designed and implemented at Ohio State with funding support from the National Fund for Medical Education. That program was intended to assess needs for educational expertise among house staff in Medicine, Obstetrics and Gynecology, Pediatrics, and Surgery, and to develop and implement a training program to improve teaching skills. Dr. Briggs was the former chief surgical resident who participated in the pilot house staff training program.

Initially that program was designed to permit each resident several opportunities to become familar with instructional skills useful in planning, presenting, and evaluating a clinical teaching session. Opportunities to develop specific teaching skills were provided through microteaching experiences distributed over several weeks. An important part of the microteaching experience was that of receiving feedback relative to preplanned or impromptu videotaped sessions, and developing skills in instructional observation and evaluation. Program objectives were keyed to specified teaching activities where the participating departments' house staff worked through the program independently and at their own pace.

The pilot program was extremely labor intensive and was discontinued for lack of funding, but Dr. Briggs's experience in that program was positive. He helped sustain interest in developing a new program. The major differences between the proposed house staff teaching skills program and the previous pilot program were our experience and the necessity of planning for a program of narrower scope because of limited resources, a program that was both efficient and effective.

Two factors contributed to the Department of Surgery's renewed interest in developing a house staff teaching skills program: the recent success in the Department of Medicine, and Dr. Briggs's and the division's link to past house staff teaching skills development efforts.

Working with the Undergraduate Education Committee

The Undergraduate Education Committee invited us to discuss ways to improve the teaching skills of surgical residents. Although the committee realized we had worked with other departments, most recently with the Department of Medicine, they wanted to emphasize that teaching in surgery has unique qualities. Told that surgery was different from other specialties, we encouraged the faculty to suspend initial claims of uniqueness and simply explore a number of key questions for planning purposes. We assured them that as discussions progressed they would have every opportunity to alter an evolving program should Surgery's special needs be overlooked.

Three questions guided our initial discussions. Accepting that knowledge of surgery and clinical competence were needed, we asked, "What kinds of training do you think surgical residents need in order to prepare them for teaching? What responsibilities do residents have for teaching medical students, other house staff, and faculty? Given the following settings for teaching—ward rounds, grand rounds, noon conferences, morbidity/mortality conferences, teaching in the operating room—in what aspects of teaching do residents need training and assistance?" Discussion was lively and enthusiastic during the meeting. At the conclusion all agreed that work should begin on planning an ongoing teaching skills training program. The group decided that a planning team, including Dr. Briggs, two surgery division chiefs, and the chief resident, would work with us to develop the program.

The planning team met regularly to discuss several issues: whom to include, methods of delivery, content to be covered, and means for seminar evaluation. For us an important adjunct to the planning discussions was to observe directly resident and faculty teaching activities.

Observing Surgery Teaching Activities

We were invited by department chiefs, residents, and medical students to attend and to observe the daily events on the hospital wards; in the operating rooms; at teaching, work, and grand rounds; and at various staff conferences. Our belief was that we could not present ourselves as credible members of the seminar teaching team without direct observation experience.

Four division staff members observed various surgery-teaching activities. More than 140 total hours of observations were recorded by the four professional educators. In addition to morning rounds, some of us scrubbed for surgery and watched thoracic, gastrointestinal, plastic, and orthopedic surgery. We observed how attending physicians demonstrated teaching. Our concern was to be attentive to the teachable moment or lack of teaching in the operating room. Clearly, if things were going well during a procedure, the attending physician was able to do much more deliberate teaching than if things were going "poorly." We considered these observations an essential part of our seminar planning. As educators, we had several questions in mind as we observed surgery residents teaching. Some of the questions were:

1. What are the residents' expectations of the medical students they teach? How have they organized their teaching?
2. Did surgery residents spend much time with students in one-to-one instruction? How about conferences or in small-group settings?
3. Did residents capitalize on "teachable moments" during work rounds?
4. Was the rumor true that the best teaching opportunities occurred in the evening hours?
5. What unique teaching occurred in operating rooms during surgery? What opportunities were missed?

In a way, our observations generated background material for planning the seminar. We used our observational notes as a way to record interesting vignettes concerning teaching. Some were good examples, and some were not. We wanted to have specific examples of surgical instruction that we could use during the seminar to highlight particular points. We wanted to try to "speak the language" of the surgical resident. The observations, however, were not planned as a field study of surgery teaching. We did not try to specify and then categorize classes of teaching successes and failures. Our main observations were intended chiefly to confirm the existence of some general principles of clinical teaching with which we were already familar, and to acquaint ourselves with specific examples of surgery teaching and teaching contexts.

At first our observations were rather general. We noted the variety of ways house officers received and presented clinical instructions while providing patient-care services. As observers, we did not try to hide our presence. Students often assumed we were physicians. When we scrubbed for surgery, some assumed we were part of the surgical team. Most persons welcomed our presence on the wards and in the operating room. When the opportunity presented itself, we introduced ourselves as medical educators interested in observing how teaching is done in surgery.

We especially wanted to observe and document good process skills of teaching, such as asking questions that required more than a simple recall of facts. Some residents seemed to be good at teaching, whereas others were poor.

> One day we had rounded in the surgery intensive care unit (SICU) with a team composed of a senior resident, an intern, and three third- year medical students. The students were in the second month of their 2-month surgery clerkship. Just outside the patient area of the SICU, the house officers and students were reading charts and the resident asked, "What is the significance of having a temperature spike on a patient presenting with the following (charted) symptoms?"

This was an excellent open-ended question. The students responded with a variety of calculated guesses. We later compared the question with one offered by another resident.

> Dr. Emily Smith, a senior surgical resident, asked one of her three medical students to pick up the chart. "Who has the patient in 716?" "I do," answered Tom, and he began to present the case. "Wait a second," said Emily. "What's the most common complication of Meckel's diverticulum in adults?"

Such closed-ended questions, although relevant to patient care, do not provide the student with an opportunity to think critically or to practice problem-solving. For us the concern was with the context in which the question was posed. With Dr. Smith's question, we were uncertain, and Tom's expression suggested similar confusion. Examples like these were ones we documented as we tried to gain an understanding of the residents' current teaching styles.

The students on surgery were especially helpful. On one occasion we held a 30-minute "debriefing session" with 40 third-year medical students just completing their 2-month clinical rotation in surgery. We asked the students several questions about the nature and scope of teaching during the clerkship: Who does the teaching? What was helpful or effective instruction? What was ineffective instruction? What guidance and feedback did they (the students) receive? What instructional behaviors and patterns would they like to see changed, continued, and/or modified? Generally the students wanted "meaningful" time. As Anne put it, "There is no learning that takes place when I spend 3 hours in surgery on the end of a retractor."

Again, we took notes on our observations. These we used to help focus our planning for the teaching skills seminar. As it turned out, there were many issues related to education in surgery that needed attention. Many fell outside the scope of teaching surgery residents to teach. Rather than ignore these other important educational issues, we planned to incorporate some discussion of the issues in the seminar. Of the number of concerns and issues about teaching that emerged from our observations, the main ones were as follows:

1. We noted that surgery was a discipline that induced mastery of motor skills. Although all residents do teach basic procedures to medical students, we believed that some emphasis on the teaching of procedures would benefit surgical residents particularly.

2. From our observations we concluded that the concept of a teacher-as-manager was a useful way to characterize the residents' challenge to manage a team of learners having diverse learning needs. We had also noted that a resident's team might include interns, third- and fourth-year medical students, fellows, faculty, nurses, and nursing students. We eventually decided to focus on the teaching of undergraduate medical students, but our observations reminded us that residents teach many different levels of learners. Teaching and managing a small group of students turned out to be an important resident teaching skill.

3. We observed that most residents would be called on to present lectures occasionally. We therefore were sure to consider presenting a segment on effective lecture skills.

4. We noted that many department educational policies were either unclear or not enforced. For example, many residents were not sure where medical students were supposed to be and when. We learned that there was ambiguity about roles and responsibilities for teaching and learning. Furthermore, we realized that we could not address all the concerns about departmental education policy during the seminar, but we thought faculty in the department should address these matters.

5. Perhaps the most interesting observation was that many of the

residents intuitively performed well as teachers. One of our hopes for the seminar was to reinforce their commonsense teaching habits.

The observations were useful in several ways. We gained firsthand experience with the teaching problems and possibilities presented in surgery. We came to appreciate a number of educational issues that had an impact on surgery instruction, and we became recognized as medical educators interested in surgery instruction. By the time the seminar was presented, observation and planning had spanned 6 months.

IMPLEMENTING THE TEACHING SKILLS SEMINAR

Surgical rounds provided us with more than a base on which to organize a house staff teaching skills seminar. In retrospect, the experience of going on rounds gave us a Gestalt conception of the busy resident and the teaching hospital, and an appreciation of the hectic schedules maintained by house staff. Understanding the surgery teaching environment was important to our planning if we had any hopes of succeeding with the seminar.

Several key questions guided the planning process: Should we plan a performance-based teaching skills program or an awareness-oriented program? What presentation formats should we use? How much outside reading should we assign, if any? These questions were discussed during several meetings with the surgery planning team, key house staff, and our professional education colleagues within the Division of Research and Evaluation in Medical Education.

Eventually we decided that a successful first program must be a fast-paced, 1-day seminar. The focus of the seminar was to present a practical overview of important teaching principles and process skills. There would be little time for residents to practice or get feedback on their own teaching skills; the seminar would essentially be an introductory, awareness-oriented program. Deciding that it would be as important to model good teaching as it was to tell about it, we ended up with a seminar that would cover a limited number of topics, presented in a variety of ways, that would give the residents a conceptual framework for improving their own teaching.

The tone of the seminar was informal, and residents' active participation in discussions of teaching was encouraged. As a result of the seminar, we expected surgery residents to increase their awareness of (1) fundamental principles of clinical teaching, (2) the variety of individual teaching styles, (3) specific skills used in giving feedback to students, providing small-group instruction, and teaching procedural or psychomotor skills, and (4) Department of Surgery educational policy issues.

So that all residents could attend one of four identical sessions, schedules were arranged by the chief surgical resident and division chiefs. Logistically, it was convenient that the Division of General Surgery devoted 1 day per week to meetings and medical education activities. Thus it was reasonable to schedule one of the seminars on a Thursday and another on a Saturday, with repeat performances the following week.

The seminar was presented four times in July, shortly after the arrival of newly appointed surgical house officers. Repeating the seminar four times guaranteed adequate ward coverage and kept seminar groups to a manageable size. A total of 66 residents attended one of the four seminars, held off-campus and away from the distractions of the hospital. Having about 14 residents present at any one session assured us that opportunities for individual participation and involvement would be high.

To further insulate the residents from their patient-care responsibilities, we arranged for the residents to check in their beepers at the door. One staff person was responsible throughout the day for taking all beeper calls. Urgent messages were then relayed to the residents.

Once the logistics were worked out, we felt confident that the sessions would be helpful. The 8-hour seminar was designed to increase residents' awareness of important educational problems, possibilities, and responsibilities.

Seminar Content, Materials, and Teaching Faculty

A key decision by the planning team was to have professional educators from the division provide most of the instruction during the seminar. Table 11.1 outlines the seminar agenda.

Four professional educators from the division presented one or more components of the program. The major topics presented were:

Principles of Good Teaching—This 40-minute session presented an overview of key components of effective teaching: establishing goals and expectations for the student, motivating the student, stimulating the student's memory, directing the student's attention, communicating with the student, providing appropriate practice, and evaluating and reinforcing the student (Schwenk and Whitman, 1984; Stritter and Flair, 1980).

Effective Feedback Skills—This small-group session provided for a discussion and definition of effective feedback skills for educational development of students and as an important preface to evaluation (Ende, 1983).

Effective Lecture Skills—This session described the characteristics of a good lecture (Foley and Smilansky, 1980).

Small-Group Teaching Skills—This lecture-discussion session outlined key problems and solutions found in small-group teaching settings (Dutton et al., 1972; Prater and Laputz, 1984).

Skills of Teaching Procedures—This small-group session provided opportunity for analysis of technical skills teaching and definition of a model for teaching psychomotor skills (Barrett, 1984; Bell, 1984).

Three components of the seminar were presented to the entire group:

Principles, Lecturing, and Small-Group Teaching

Two small-group, skill-acquisition sessions were held simultaneously with half the total group. One small-group session addressed the need for providing timely, accurate, and corrective feedback to learners. The other focused on ways to teach procedural skills to students properly. Residents later switched groups so that by day's end the entire group had experienced both small-group sessions. As noted earlier, in the planning we decided to eliminate microteaching-type segments in the program. Time did not permit adequate opportunity for microteaching analysis and feedback. It also seemed logical to consider incorporating such an approach in future seminars or using it for residents identified for remediation of poor teaching habits. In an all-encompassing approach like this seminar, covering a range of topics essential to clinical teaching before analyzing individuals' strengths and weaknesses seemed more appropriate.

Throughout the seminar a strategy of the teaching team was to model good teaching and various teaching methods. The session on teaching procedures was but one example of the way we tried to introduce a variety of teaching methods and the importance of variety in teaching. In an early planning session, one author (JP) described his lesson plan for the procedures segment.

> After briefly introducing the topic I'll ask the whole group to take 5 minutes to brainstorm a list of procedures that residents often need to teach medical students. These will be listed by one of the residents on a chalkboard as the others call out examples. From the list I'll point out nasogastric intubation as the procedure we will use as an example throughout the ses-

TABLE 11.1 Department of Surgery House Staff Teaching-Skills Seminar Agenda July 1985

Time	Activity/topic
7:30–8:00	Coffee and doughnuts
8:00–8:10	Introductions
8:10–8:20	Purpose of seminar
8:20–8:50	Issues identification
8:50–9:30	Principles of good teaching
9:30–10:00	Training Styles Inventory (TSI)
10:00–11:00	Skills session*
11:00–11:45	Lecture skills
11:45–12:15	Resident reactions
12:15–1:00	Lunch
1:00–2:00	Skills session*
2:00–3:00	Small-group teaching skills
3:00–3:15	TSI results and recapitulation
3:15–3:45	Department education policy
3:45–4:00	Seminar evaluation
4:00	Adjourn

*Skills Sessions: "Feedback and Communication Skills" and "Teaching Procedures."

sion. It is a common procedure that we can dissect for the purpose of identifying important steps in teaching psychomotor skills. Next, I'll announce that I need two volunteers. Then I'll have all residents take pencil and paper and plot step-by-step how each would plan and conduct effective teaching of nasogastric intubation. Next the two volunteers will orally and through role play demonstrate how each would teach a naive student how to pass an NG tube. After the volunteers finish, we will critique each and discuss the underlying instructional strategy used for teaching this procedure. I will next present a model for effectively teaching psychomotor skills (for example, orient the student, demonstrate, instructor talk-through, student talk-through, and student practice). Next I will show a videotape of nasogastric intubation that we will critique according to the model. Finally we will discuss the practical limitations (like time and access to patients) on using the model in all cases.

The above example included participation by the residents as a way to circumvent their passivity. Various audiovisual methods were used, including videotape of the procedure, listing of topics on the chalkboard, overhead projection of the model, and handouts. All were used within the hour set aside for the session. We wanted to introduce the residents to the many instructional possibilities that exist for their use. Throughout the seminar we called attention to the pacing and methods we used, so that the residents might begin to recognize instructional process as well as principles.

As part of the seminar, each resident received a packet of materials for his future reference. The packet included handouts related to each presentation, a teaching-style self-assessment instrument, a seminar evaluation form, and a listing of references and resources. The handouts were described, used, or identified during the seminar, so that the residents would have something for future use.

The final session of the seminar was not a skills-oriented session, but rather one devoted to identification of education-related policy issues that affected the residents. Examples of their concerns about educational policies in surgery were: What incentives can be offered to encourage good teaching? What can we (residents) legitimately expect of students? What are the attending physicians' roles in teaching medical students? When will we get feedback on our teaching strengths and weaknesses? Should medical students be required to be in the hospital after 6:00 P.M.? These examples represented some of the issues that affected the residents' abilities to carry out their teaching responsibilities. Clearly, the issues were not going to be resolved during the seminar, but faculty members present at the seminar and the residents found it useful to have the education-related policy issues listed and discussed.

EVALUATING THE TEACHING-SKILLS SEMINAR

Residents completed seminar evaluations at the end of the seminar. The evaluation form asked questions falling under two general categories: residents' reactions to the content of the seminar (e.g., teaching skills) and residents' perceptions of the seminar format. Residents responded to 12 items on the basis of their reactions to the seminar. A three-response category (not helpful, somewhat helpful, very helpful) was used for six questions. Five questions used a Likert-type response set. One item was open-ended and asked for comments. Responses were held in strict confidence, tallied, and reported as group data to the Undergraduate Education Committee.

In general, most residents reported an increased interest in teaching as a result of the seminar. Eighty-five percent ($N = 57$) either agreed or strongly agreed that the seminar stimulated their interest in teaching. Seventy-seven percent ($N = 51$) reported that they would be willing to participate in future sessions devoted to improving teaching.

Reactions to the quality of seminar instruction were equally favorable. Eighty-eight percent of the residents ($N = 58$) either agreed or strongly agreed that seminar topics were presented effectively. Ninety-one percent ($N = 60$) reported that the seminar was "of some value" or "definitely valuable" as a learning experience. Still, most thought the seminar was "too long" (55%, $N = 35$). Forty-five percent ($N = 29$) thought the length of the seminar was "about right."

A disappointment noted by many residents in their written remarks was that attending physicians were not required to participate in such a session. The other few negative remarks indicated a perception that the seminar was a "waste of time." However, they nearly all indicated a favorable reaction to the program. As one resident put it, "I enjoyed the day. The main advantage of this session was to focus on the need for all of us (residents and faculty) to concentrate on the teaching process. The chance to interact with other residents was stimulating, and we need more opportunities to do this." Overall, the seminar evaluations suggested that the teaching skills seminar was a successful first step in the Department of Surgery's efforts to upgrade the education program for students.

CONCLUSIONS AND RECOMMENDATIONS

We end every training program with one question: "Where do we go from here?" We want to invoke the same question here. We believed our efforts to plan and implement a teaching skills seminar for residents were adequate at the time. Perhaps if we were to plan the surgery program anew we might do things differently. For now, we have these recommendations for others who might be planning a teaching skills seminar for surgical house staff:

- Have a group of faculty physicians, residents, students, and professional educators plan jointly a teaching skills program.
- Have professional educators round with residents to identify patterns of teaching and to gain an understanding of residents' perceptions of teaching in the local context.
- Determine whether the needs for teaching skills are uniform for residents in general surgery and the subspecialties. Is the length of time residents have with students important? Some surgical specialties see students for only 2 weeks, whereas general surgery might see the same students for a month.

Experience has provided valuable lessons and greater understanding of the role of the house staff in teaching medical students. At the Ohio State University College of Medicine we have learned these lessons:

- Teaching is third on the list of residents' priorities, following patient care and their own professional development (and survival!).
- There is no ideal schedule for arranging teaching skills seminars. Residents' perceptions of time and responsibilities will always run contrary to any scheduling plans.
- One should recognize from the outset that teaching is an unfamiliar practice and responsibility for residents.
- Faculty inactivity in the teaching enterprise can be a barrier to producing a successful program for improving residents' teaching skills.

These recommendations present no surprises. As professionals in education, we have found that often a good teacher differs from a bad one by the fact that the former cares about students and their learning. We believe, however, that it is important to continue drawing attention to clinical teaching and its unique problems and challenging possibilities. Clinical teaching can truly be an exciting experience and perhaps is the best way to learn.

Where have we gone from there? Although we offered personal consulting to any resident requesting assistance in teaching, we were not surprised that none of these busy house staff has called. This is not a failing as much as it reflects the reality of a life situation; surgery faculty and residents have multiple responsibilities, only one of which is to teach. However, we have noticed some progress related to our seminar efforts. For instance, we have helped the department redesign its resident-evaluation procedures. And recently, we were invited by Dr. Briggs to develop four educational grand rounds for the Department of Surgery. And as of this writing, we have just completed another clinical teaching skills seminar for newly arriving, first-year surgical residents.

CHAPTER 12

Teaching Medicine Residents to Teach

MARTHA G. CAMP
J. DENNIS HOBAN

In 1983 Wake Forest University's Bowman Gray School of Medicine offered its first organized program for instructing residents in how to teach. The program was presented at North Carolina Baptist Hospital, our affiliated residency training hospital. We identified four main reasons for developing teaching skills in residents. First, the education of medical students and more "junior" residents, as derived from daily encounters with the house staff, could be enhanced. Second, the teaching that residents provide for their patients and to the medical staff could be improved. Third, the course could develop skills needed in later community leadership roles. And fourth, interest in careers in academic medicine might well be engendered by the course.

In developing our particular course, we chose objectives that addressed only some of these potential outcomes. Had circumstances allowed for a longer course, a great deal more might have been included. We believed, though, that the residents should leave the course with the sense that they would like to know more about teaching rather than with the feeling of having touched superficially on all the potential topics. Therefore, the specific objectives of the course were limited by time constraints to only the most pressing instructional needs. Those needs were linked to the fact that our medical school, as do most, places the burden of clinical teaching on the house officer.

The expected outcomes of our course were that the participating residents would:

1. Gain knowledge of educational principles and practices that could be applied to their hospital/medical school setting.
2. Become familiar with some of the research literature related to teaching practices in medical education.
3. Use important educational principles in at least one type of teaching session.

PLANNING THE COURSE

What we had hoped to do with this first course was to show evidence that it could comfortably be taken in spite of the time constraints in residency programs and that there would be clearly observable benefits. Thus, this first course might be considered a pilot of what could be done to enhance teaching skills of residents.

Selection of Instructors

This course had its origin in a brief discussion between two faculty members—a young clinician and an educational specialist. The clinician had a strong interest in teaching, had recently completed both medical school and residency training at our institution, and was eager to improve teaching at the graduate level.

The course evolved as a collaborative effort of doctoral-level medical educators along with clinicians in a residency training program—two physicians in the Department of Internal Medicine and two faculty members in the Office of Educational Research and Services. This particular combination brought together an appropriate mix of educational expertise and clinical credibility, so that the course could be planned and taught with optimum efficiency and effectiveness. A medical school rarely has faculty members trained in both medicine and education to design and teach such a course. Thus, our use of a combination of faculty with differing areas of expertise approximated the ideal. In addition to training in clinical medicine or education, those who taught the course were perceived as good teachers by the residents. This was important for establishing the credibility of the instructors in this first course on teaching.

Selection of Department

In selecting the clinical department to be involved in our first resident-teaching course, we wanted one whose faculty and department head expressed interest. We chose the Department of Medicine, the academic "home" of our clinical instructors and a department that offered solid administrative support and funding.

Selection of Students

Sixteen soon-to-be-third-year house officers in internal medicine were invited to participate in the course. About three-fourths of those invited chose to participate, and all of those completed the course. The homogeneity of the group in terms of common clinical experience and similar teaching responsibilities had three advantages. First, because the participants knew one another, we did not need to devise activities during the course to develop the trust essential to open discussion. Second, because of their familiarity with one another, participants were more at ease in exchanging accounts of their own teaching experiences. Finally, the residents were able to provide constructive criticism to one another as they observed each other both in the course itself and in clinical teaching settings. The atmosphere, then, was one of free and open exchange.

The Logistical Realities

If residency programs required that each new resident be taught how to be an effective teacher, then courses such as ours would be in great demand. The reality, however, is much more likely to be that one or two faculty members in a residency training program will show a willingness to approach their chairman with a proposal for a teacher-development program, and their chairman will agree to at least let them try it. Such was our case. Our course was voluntary, not for credit, but carried the backing of the department chairman.

We believed that in designing a course we needed to be as considerate as possible of the time and energy demands on the residents. In our program, we scheduled the sessions to be held from 5:00 P.M. till 7:00 P.M. in a room adjacent to the hospital. We provided a light dinner for the participants, paid for by funds from the residents' department.

Because house officers frequently work long hours, we had to find a time at which they could all assemble. Given during the dinner hour once a week for 4 weeks, our course seldom interfered with their other work responsibilities and did not greatly extend their workday.

DEVELOPING THE COURSE

Planning the Overall Strategy

The four course developers/instructors held a series of meetings to develop course objectives, an outline, teaching materials, and strategies. Once the overall plan was developed, we also met after each session to talk about the impact of the session on the residents, to assess/evaluate the activities used, and to plan the specifics of the next session.

As part of the planning process, we reviewed the relevant literature, beginning with material specific to medical education, extending into that of other health professions, and finally into the general areas of learning and teaching. Especially helpful were the data from a survey two of us had conducted of Offices of Medical Education at U.S. medical schools (Hoban and Camp, 1980), which provided a wealth of materials used by other medical educators in similar settings. The educational specialists of our team reviewed and screened all of the instructional materials obtained as a result of that survey for their potential usefulness in our course. Those materials that seemed the most promising were later reviewed by our clinical colleagues.

Deciding what to teach also depended on our personal observations of residents at work. For the medical education specialists of the teaching team, it was important to have firsthand knowledge of the residents' teaching and clinical care responsibilities and how they were being carried out. We therefore spent considerable time observing ward rounds, case conferences, grand rounds, and other scheduled and spontaneous educational settings. Each of the educational-specialist instructors attended at least two ward rounds, two case conferences, and two grand rounds during the month preceding the course. We took note of typical and atypical teaching strategies used, opportunities for teaching, and the persons who did the teaching in various settings. During the sessions of our course, we were then able to refer to real situations in which we had observed the residents and others engaged in teaching. We used them as concrete examples of appropriate and inappropriate teaching behaviors.

Organizing Each Session and Assigning Teaching Responsibilities

Our first task was to identify the teaching settings that residents encounter.

Our list included:

1. Case presentations (e.g., at mortality conferences)

2. Teaching on rounds (e.g., of more junior residents and of medical students)
3. Teaching clinical skills in the medical school course on physical diagnosis and in clinical clerkships
4. Making large-group presentations (lectures), such as grand rounds and departmental conferences

Our overall strategy for the course was to address each of these teaching situations with some didactic material along with out-of-class readings, written exercises, and, where possible, instruction using various media. Also, in each session we provided opportunity for concrete, "hands-on" practical experience, such as teaching a novice how to take a blood pressure reading. As instructors, we attempted to model those teaching behaviors we were hoping the residents would acquire.

Assessing Results and Revising the Course

We planned from the outset to solicit comments and other feedback from our students, both formally, in writing, and informally, in "hallway consults." Changes and improvements in our later programs resulted directly from this feedback. Those course components that worked well were retained; those that did not were modified for the next course. Not only was this good instructional design technique, but it increased participant enthusiasm for the course because they believed that their feedback was important.

IMPLEMENTATION

Having planned the course, the instructors scheduled four instructional sessions for the residents. Each session lasted 2 hours and included a light meal and beverage. Each instructor took major responsibility for one of the sessions, and the other three were present to help elaborate and embellish the session topic or to facilitate small groups. Each session is described below in terms of rationale, teaching materials, and teaching/learning strategies.

Session I: Introduction to Clinical Teaching

A. Complete *Clinical Supervision: A Written Simulation*
B. Discuss teaching roles of clinical supervisors
C. Handouts

(McMaster University, 1981; Reuler et al.; 1982)

A warm-up for the course, Session I began with a meal and informal chat about the events of the day. Then an overview of the total course was given and our expectations for the residents as participants in the course were described. Our intent was to start the residents thinking seriously about what teaching was all about, so, after the initial overview, a clinical faculty member asked the residents to complete a written simulation developed by the Association of American Medical Colleges entitled *Clinical Supervision.* The setting of the simulation is as follows:

> You are a clinical preceptor responsible for supervising medical students toward the end of their "Introduction to Clinical Medicine" course, just prior to beginning their first clinical clerkship. This morning you will work with Jim Scott, who will be doing his first complete new-patient workup. The other day you heard . . . that the student is "something of a dud." Your tasks today are to evaluate his performance, to give him feedback, and to arrange whatever follow-up instruction you feel is appropriate. . . . You and Jim greet each other and begin to plan the morning's activities. (Association of American Medical Colleges, 1976)

At this point the residents were asked to decide what they would say to Jim Scott. The simulation then proceeded through a number of decisions that the resident needs to work through as a teacher. Although no decision-making paths through the simulation were definitely wrong, some paths were certainly preferable to others.

The path chosen by each resident was explored and discussed. The discussion was subdued, but it helped the residents to focus on the fact that in the teaching/learning process a teacher must choose specific courses of action. The simulation, however, was not as satisfactory an opening strategy as we had hoped it would be. The participants seemed to have little enthusiasm for the simulation, and no general principles of the teaching/learning process emerged. Perhaps the proper placement for such a simulation exercise is later in the course, after the residents have thought more about clinical teaching.

Session II: Large-Group Presentations

A. Lecture on "lecturing"
B. Review specific guidelines
C. Discuss good and poor examples
D. Handouts

(Giles et al., 1982; Maddox and Hoole, 1975; Stuart and Rutherford, 1978; Thomas, 1972; Whitman, 1983)

This session was essentially a lecture about lecturing, modeling appropriate techniques. It began with a description of the lecture method, its weaknesses and strengths, and a synopsis of the research that has been done on the lecture as a teaching technique.

The remainder of the session focused on "how-to" guidelines for preparing, organizing, and delivering a lecture and using audiovisual materials. These topics are outlined in Table 12.1.

Session III: Informal Teaching

A. View *G. Patton, M.D.* videotape (Fidler and Alexander, 1979)
B. Discuss teaching styles
C. Discuss helpful teacher behaviors
D. Handouts
(Daggett et al., 1979; Stritter et al., 1975; Tremonti and Biddle, 1982)

Session III began with a videotape entitled *G. Patton, M.D.,* obtained from the Health Sciences Consortium. This tape depicted the "Patton" style of teaching medicine, i.e., dogmatic, authoritarian, combative. After the videotape, a clinician led a discussion of the style that Patton portrayed. Some residents identified the Pattons they had met in medical education. The group leader than helped the residents identify those stylistic components of Patton that could be helpful in some situations as well as those that might be destructive.

After reviewing teaching styles, the residents then examined a study on teacher behaviors thought to be useful for fourth-year medical students (Stritter et al., 1975). The instructor was careful to explain that the study did not "prove" that the teacher behaviors caused learning, but rather that students believed that certain teacher behaviors were helpful in the teaching/learning process. That study was used to indicate the difficulty in knowing how teaching and learning relate.

The residents seemed to respond openly and enthusiastically, most of them reporting having encountered a "Patton" and all of them admitting that they had well-formed opinions about what good teachers do.

Session IV: Teaching the Novice

A. View *Fingerweaving* videotape
B. Demonstrate examination of the abdomen
C. Review model for teaching psychomotor skills
D. Handout
(Yelon, 1973)

TABLE 12.1 Guidelines for Preparing, Organizing, and Delivering a Lecture and Using Audiovisual Materials

Preparing a lecture

A. Be aware of time restrictions
B. Define learner needs
C. Determine information learnable per unit time
D. Outline the content
E. Practice your presentation

Organizing a lecture

A. Introduction
1. Gain attention
2. Relate to something known
3. State the purpose
4. State learning objectives
5. Motivate

B. Body
1. Start with problem or series of questions
2. Use examples
3. Compare and/or contrast ideas
4. Summarize frequently
5. Make clear transitions between teaching points

C. Conclusion
1. Summarize
2. Suggest ways of using material

Delivering the lecture

A. Appearance
1. Make good eye contact
2. Use meaningful movements
3. Be conscious of distracting gestures

B. Voice
1. Vary your pitch
2. Vary your volume
3. Vary your rate

C. Attitude
1. Be helpful
2. Be businesslike
3. Use natural humor
4. Answer questions, if possible

Use audiovisual methods when they:

1. Help clarify the subject
2. Are appropriate to the subject matter
3. Increase interest in the subject matter
4. Save time
5. Help students remember

This session began with the viewing of a videotape, *Fingerweaving.* Produced at the Medical University of South Carolina, it shows clearly how the viewpoints of a demonstration differ for the instructor and for the student. It also shows the importance of reducing a complex procedure to small, easy-to-learn steps.

A model for teaching physical examination skills and procedures to beginning students was then explained and demonstrated. A guest instructor, a senior faculty member, used that instructional model to teach one of the educational-specialist instructors how to examine the abdomen properly. The model for such teaching (from Yelon, 1973) is shown in Table 12.2.

REVISIONS IN LATER PROGRAMS

The time, location, and level of course presentation seemed to be appropriate and were maintained in later courses. However, the course directors thought that some parts of the course should be altered in subsequent offerings. A major change was the replacement of the AAMC educational simulation. The educational simulation session might

TABLE 12.2 Model for Teaching Psychomotor Skills

A psychomotor skill is a physical skill; it involves the use of muscles in a smooth, precise, well-timed performance. The skill is organized to relate to the space around the individual, and the skill is timed so that each muscle comes into play in consort with other muscles at specific points in the sequence of given activities. Examples: writing, drawing, operating machinery or laboratory equipment, swimming, sewing, driving.

Phases in teaching psychomotor skills

I. Introductory	II. Practice	III. Perfecting
A. prepare student for learning the skill	A. require practice of the skill	A. require precision in performance
B. provide information about the skill	B. observe student practice, and prompt when needed	B. observe and prompt on details
C. analyze the skill	C. provide feedback when needed	C. provide feedback on fine points

have been effective had it been placed later in the course, rather than at the beginning. Instead, we elected to drop it. In its place we used the provocative videotape *G. Patton, M.D.* Because this videotape generates discussion about teaching styles and teacher effectiveness, it provided an excellent beginning for our next course on teaching. In the place of the session on informal teaching, we then developed a session on effective case presentations, based on feedback from residents in our first course that this skill has high priority for them.

Our case presentation session took the approach that for residents to teach others to present cases properly, they need to be able to *model* good presentations. The class was divided into two groups, each with a clinician instructor as well as a medical education specialist instructor to provide immediate feedback to the residents. After simulations of a "good" and a "bad" presentation by the clinician instructor, each resident presented a short case to the group. Table 12.3 illustrates the rating scale used by all participants while observing the short case presentations.

EVALUATION OF THE COURSE

Because the course was for a small group of participants and was a "pilot," we planned its evaluation to be simple and practical. Mainly we wanted to get a feel for the satisfaction level of the participants and to observe as each participant conducted a teaching session. We had little baseline information on how well the participants taught before the course, so we could only assume that the course had some effect on their subsequent performance. We relied on the participants' self-reports regarding their satisfaction with the course.

Assessment Questionnaire

An end-of-course questionnaire was used to assess satisfaction and perceived value of the course. All participants reported that the course was valuable and had caused them to think about new approaches to teaching. Most said they had less anxiety about teaching than they had before the course, but they were still undecided about whether they had more confidence in their ability to be good clinical teachers. All the sessions received about the same positive rating. Apparent from the questionnaire was that the faculty made the participants feel comfortable and better able to assess their strengths and weaknesses related to teaching. All participants stated that it was appropriate to have a clinician and an educational specialist as instructors. One participant com-

TABLE 12.3 Case Presentation Critique

1. Organization of material

____	____	____	____	____
poorly organized		average organization		well organized

2. Clarity of presentation

____	____	____	____	____
unclear		somewhat clear		very clear

3. Pace

____	____	____	____	____
too slow		about right		too fast

4. Eye contact

____	____	____	____	____
poor		average		excellent

5. Length

____	____	____	____	____
too short		about right		too long

6. Quality of information

____	____	____	____	____
too much irrelevant information		some relevant/ some irrelevant information		very pertinent information

Comments

mented that "nonmedicine people can make comments more objectively . . . and a medical person provides connection to practical aspects of teaching."

Observation of Teaching

For a period of several months after the course sessions were completed, an instructor observed each participant as he or she conducted a teaching session. For the most part, the observations were of formal lectures or of case presenations. The observer/instructor looked for evidence of the use of "good" or "poor" presentation techniques and then provided feedback to each resident on these points after the teaching session. The feedback tended to be positive and reinforced those aspects of their presentations that the residents had done well. By and large, the faculty observers believed that the participants showed that they had put into practice many of the skills that had been discussed and demonstrated in the course on teaching, particularly skills in organizing material, generating audience involvement, developing handouts, and summarizing and emphasizing important points.

Cost Analysis

In any education program, it is important to be aware of costs. Although a cost/benefit analysis in a human services area such as teaching is difficult to conduct because the measures of outcomes are generally subjective, we could at least estimate whether the costs of such services were reasonable.

In our analysis we asked some basic questions and drew some conclusions. Our questions related to how much money was expended to conduct the course and whether there are alternative training programs that should be considered in light of the cost analysis.

We concluded that using four instructors for the course was not necessary for the course to be effective. On the other hand, each of the instructors would gain valuable experience by participating for the first time in this type of course.

Also, only limited performance objectives would be met as a result of such a short course. Students would have to practice their skills beyond the course if they were to improve their teaching behaviors significantly.

Given the assumptions of the cost analysis and the limited number of participating students, it was necessary to find a simple method for determining whether the course had been developed and implemented at a reasonable cost to the institution. We came up with a determination of costs for faculty (planning and teaching time) and for supplies (food, instructional materials, audiovisual equipment expenses, photocopying, and miscellaneous costs).

We calculated that our course cost less than $1,000 and were pleased to find that it was less than the sum that would be required to bring in outside consultants as course developers/instructors. Institutionally, this is an important finding because it keeps dollar resources within the school. Furthermore, although four instructors participated in the preliminary course, when instructors work in teams of two in later courses with other audiences within the institution, the costs should be even less.

SUMMARY

We developed and taught a course for house officers on "how to teach." Two internal medicine clinicians and two medical education specialists were the original course developers and instructors; third-year residents in internal medicine were our first students. Later, other groups and other levels of residents were taught an improved version of this four 2-hour sessions course by teams of one clinician and one medical education specialist. Satisfaction has been high, and requests for additional sessions have been received from past participants.

CHAPTER **13**

Integrating Teaching and Patient Care

FRANKLIN MEDIO
LUANN WILKERSON
LINDA LESKY
STEVEN BORKAN

The importance of the resident as a clinical teacher is unquestionable. Second- and third-year residents are charged with the day-to- day supervision and instruction of first-year residents (interns) and medical students. Residents oversee clinical case management, guide clinical decision-making, and provide structured teaching activities.

The model for impromptu teaching of a procedure, examination, or other activity in the clinical setting has traditionally been "see one, do one, teach one." This model has fostered the notion that, by virtue of a medical education, residents have acquired the skills necessary for effective teaching. Unfortunately, the resident who is unskilled at teaching often fails to recognize opportunities for teaching in the educationally rich clinical environment. Instead, he gives silent attention to patient-care details during work rounds, relies excessively on medical textbooks and conference room lectures, and emphasizes inordinately the mastering of mechanical skills in providing learning experiences for interns and students.

To better prepare residents for their teaching role, the Director of

Residency Training in the Department of Medicine at Michael Reese Hospital and Medical Center in Chicago recommended that a course on teaching be started. Two of us (FM, LW) designed and offered a pilot course on clinical teaching for primary-care medical residents in the summer of 1983. Although the didactic, theoretical portions of the course were poorly received, a final session in which residents participated in a practice teaching exercise was evaluated by them as useful.

During this same time, the interns in the Department of Medicine grew increasingly dissatisfied with the lack of teaching by residents. In light of the pilot course and these complaints, we educators (FM, LW) and physicians (SB, LL) joined our intentions to revise the course. We physician faculty members served to validate for house staff the importance of teaching and provided a personal-experience perspective on resident teaching responsibilities.

To better understand how residents meet their teaching responsibilities, we observed their teaching during work rounds. The rounds were chosen as the focus for the study because they represented a daily, structured encounter between a resident, an intern, and a student for purposes of patient care. Any teaching in this setting was the resident's responsibility inasmuch as no attending physician was present.

Our observations showed that residents did not often intentionally use daily patient encounters for teaching. When they did intend to teach during work rounds, they usually provided a brief lecture. Not only did the study show the limited repertoire of teaching skills used by most residents, but it also delineated the many teaching opportunities that were being overlooked. For most residents, teaching had become synonymous with prepared lectures and was, therefore, incompatible with the unpredictable demands of patient care.

From our observational study, we designed a new Clinical Skills Teaching Course, selecting topics that would prompt residents to reexamine their limited definition of teaching and to develop teaching skills that could be easily incorporated into patient-care activities. The need for the residents' active participation as a means to effect learning, and the characterization of the house staff as learners, led to the selection of teaching methods for the course. Although both content and methods have changed with repeated offerings of the course, the goals of the course have remained constant: (1) to reinforce the residents' authority to teach; (2) to expand the residents' concept of teaching; (3) to provide opportunities for the practice of specific, practical teaching skills in a nonthreatening environment; and (4) to encourage skills in self-assessment and peer assessment of teaching effectiveness. Recognizing and capitalizing on teaching opportunities during daily patient care remains the recurring theme of the course.

PLANNING AND DEVELOPMENT

To find out how residents in the Department of Medicine met their teaching responsibilities, the authors observed 14 residents during work rounds for 1 month (Wilkerson et al., 1986). A total of 158 separate patient bedside visits were observed. The residents' teaching behaviors during these encounters were recorded by means of a checklist of 10 specific teaching skills developed from the work of Irby (1978a) and Stritter and Flair (1980). The behaviors included those teaching activities in which residents might engage in the course of routine patient care. Five members of the Department, including the residency director, reviewed the checklist to validate the behaviors included. During each observation, we also recorded factors judged to influence the amount of teaching provided by the resident on the team: on-call status, the number of patients on service, and the composition of the team. Three open-ended questions at the end of the checklist directed us to describe behaviorally each resident's leadership style, enthusiasm for teaching, and ability to organize rounds for teaching.

We found that residents on work rounds frequently engaged in three teaching behaviors; however, they did not capitalize on two of those behaviors to reinforce learning. In 69% of the cases, residents were seen to be modeling empathic communication and concern for patients, but the residents rarely discussed these interactions with members of the team. In 63% of the cases, the resident used the visit to verify some aspect of the history or physical examination, but in most of these cases, the resident did not use the opportunity to demonstrate skills or procedures. The most frequent way in which the residents were observed to provide purposeful teaching was by giving brief lectures on issues raised during the discussion of a particular patient. Mini-lecturing occurred in 40% of the interactions.

Four teaching behaviors were used infrequently in the observed resident/patient interactions: directing interns/students to pertinent publications (3%), commenting on their performance (11%), demonstrating a technique or skill (17%), and asking problem-solving questions (22%). Furthermore, two behaviors by the residents actually seemed to hinder teaching: exclusive, silent attention to patient charts and decision-making without involvement of the team. Nine of the 14 residents consistently used the time before entering the patient's room to scan the chart. Although verification of data by the resident is critical to patient care, omitting interns and residents from review of chart information during work rounds resulted in their mere quiet observance of the resident's actions. In addition, more than half of the residents consistently excluded the intern and student from participation in any clinical decision-making.

Seven of the residents who were observed enrolled later in the first Clinical Teaching Skills Course and completed a self-assessment questionnaire on teaching during work rounds. All indicated that work rounds were an appropriate setting for teaching, but only one was satisfied with the amount of time spent teaching. In describing ways in which they perceived themselves as teaching during rounds, they cited modeling of patient interaction, discussion of lab results, demonstrations of technical skills, and asking team members for management decisions. The residents indicated that in the course they would like to learn more about generalizing from specific cases, using problem-solving questions, giving feedback, and how to better structure work rounds for teaching. Almost all of the residents said they had received little feedback on their teaching and were unable to assess adequately their own teaching effectiveness.

Course Content

Our observations of work rounds and the precourse assessment led us to decide several things about the content of the proposed course. First, topics included in the course should encourage residents to question equating teaching only with lecturing and to introduce alternative teaching methods. Second, the course should focus on teaching skills that are easily used in the patient-care setting with minimal advance preparation. Finally, the course should emphatically identify teachable moments frequently overlooked by residents, specifically opportunities to demonstrate to, provide feedback for, ask questions of, and encourage participation in decision-making by interns and students. Three specific skills met these criteria and were selected for the course; giving feedback, organizing and giving mini-lectures, and using questions both to guide discussions and to teach clinical decision-making.

Teaching Methods

Two criteria guided our decisions concerning the most appropriate teaching methods for the course: attention to the role of meaningful ness and practice in learning, and a recognition of the nature of the house staff experience. Methods used in the course would need to engage the participants quickly in activities that they saw as meaningful to their roles as resident teachers. In addition, active practice and feedback would be required if the learning of new concepts and behaviors was to be facilitated.

The residents in the Department of Medicine had expressed an interest in expanding their expertise as teachers; however, they described themselves as chronically rushed, fatigued, and burdened with responsibility, having little time to devote to teaching. They were skeptical about the value of studying a nonmedical discipline, given the vast medical data to be mastered. In addition, as shown by our work rounds study, the house staff defined teaching as the expert delivery of content, an activity most often necessitating either advance preparation or extensive clinical experience.

To tailor the course to the needs of the residents and to facilitate learning, the course faculty deliberately minimized the duration of presentations on educational methods and theory. All didactic presentations were brief, focusing on definition of terms and the identification of specific skills to be learned. Most of each session was devoted to practice teaching in which each resident had the opportunity to teach other members of the group and to receive comments on his performance. The practice sessions simulated different teaching situations regularly encountered by residents, such as giving a mini-lecture, leading a discussion, or reviewing a case.

Each module began with a brief presentation by a course faculty member, characterizing the skill to be learned in the practice exercise. The resident group of eight was divided in half for practice teaching and supervised by a physician/educator faculty team. The residents simulated interns and students and reported on the teaching they observed. To begin the feedback process, each resident teacher assessed his own performance. Next, the other residents were asked to focus on their reactions as learners, commenting on the effectiveness of the resident teacher's methods and offering alternatives when appropriate. With each practice session, the residents became increasingly more effective at critiquing each other's performances. The faculty members facilitated the peer-feedback process and ensured that teaching skills, not medical knowledge, remained the focus of the feedback.

After the course, faculty members offered to observe each resident in a teaching activity of his choice. In this way the resident could apply skills learned in the course in a clinical setting and receive feedback individually. This emphasis on practice and self-evaluation increased the likelihood that teaching skills would develop. Furthermore, the practice-teaching and peer-critique process provided the residents with opportunities to observe, study, and practice teaching skills with less anxiety about their medical knowledge or concern about evaluation by an attending physician.

Planning for the course culminated with the preparation of a syllabus delineating the objectives of the course, the schedule for the four course modules, readings from medical and educational publications, and handouts describing the skills to be practiced and the procedures to be followed in preparing for the practice sessions (Table 13.1). Through participation in the course, we hoped that residents would become skilled in using various effective clinical teaching methods, integrating teaching with patient care, using questions to promote problem-solving, and evaluating their own teaching effectiveness. The modular design provided flexibility in scheduling and enabled us to meet the different demands and time constraints of each later group of residents.

Module 1: Effective Clinical Teaching

Although residents in training get considerable attention as to the development of good clinical judgment, their development of effective teaching skills is often neglected. In the first module, residents discuss specific teaching skills that characterize teachers whom they have admired, consider the special characteristics of learning in the clinical setting, and begin to develop skills in giving feedback.

During the first discussion on effective teachers, the group is challenged with the statement, "You cannot *not* teach," emphasizing that their own behaviors are constantly being observed by members of their clinical teams. Each encounter with an intern or student carries the potential for both intentional and unintentional teaching. Recognizing the powerful effect of role models in their own learning, the residents discuss ways to maximize their effectiveness as models. The group also discusses the impact on learning of active participation, clear statements of expectations, and feedback; the group also generates strategies for applying these principles in the clinical setting. To further explore strategies for teaching through feedback, the residents engage in a role-playing exercise based on their own experiences of receiving feedback from attending physicians. Working in pairs, the residents devise examples of effective and ineffective approaches to providing feedback, with each pair demonstrating a different principle of effective feedback (Ende, 1983). Adept at providing examples of ineffective feedback, the residents have a much more difficult time providing examples of effective feedback techniques. Such critiquing remains a central concern of the course because residents will provide feedback to one another in later practice sessions. The first session concludes with an explanation

TABLE 13.1 Modules for the Clinical Teaching Skills Course, Michael Reese Hospital, Chicago

Module	Objectives	Activities	Teaching Materials
Effective clinical teaching	1. Identify skills that characterize effective clinical teachers 2. Describe principles of learning applicable to the clinical setting 3. Demonstrate approaches to effective feedback	Discussion: memorable teachers Mini-lecture: learning Role play: giving feedback	Course syllabus *Learning in a Clinical Setting: Suggested Teaching Strategies* Wilkerson (1985) Ende (1983)
Lecturing and explaining	1. Describe the goals and components of a lecture 2. Determine methods for maximizing the effect of a lecture 3. Give a clear, interesting mini-lecture 4. Critique one's own lecture skills	Discussion: characteristics of a good lecture Mini-lecture: components of a lecture Practice teaching and peer critique: the lecture	*How to Prepare for Practice Teaching: The Lecture* Kroenke (1984) Bughman (1973)
Managing a small group discussion	1. Contrast the lecture and discussion 2. Describe the different functions that questions can serve in a discussion 3. Demonstrate techniques for facilitating discussions 4. Critique one's own discussion skills	Mini-lecture: use of questions Practice exercise: identifying the function of a question Practice teaching and peer critique: the discussion	*How to Prepare for Practice Teaching: Small Group Discussion* *Questions as a Teaching Tool* Napell (1976)

(*continued*)

TABLE 13.1 (*Continued*)

Module	Objectives	Activities	Teaching Materials
Teaching one-to-one	1. Explain how a case presentation can be used to teach 2. Demonstrate questioning techniques that foster problem-solving skills 3. Integrate modeling, feedback, and discussion in impromptu teaching	Discussion: possible goals of case-based teaching Minilecture: approaches to teaching one-to-one Practice teaching and peer critique: case presentation	*How to Prepare for Practice Teaching: One-on-one on Work and Chart Rounds* Kassirer (1983) Linfors and Neelon (1980)

of the assignment for the next session, preparing and giving a brief lecture.

Module 2: Lecturing and Explaining

Because it is the most frequently observed and most clearly accepted teaching method used by the residents, the lecture is selected as the least threatening skill with which to begin the practice teaching (see also Chapter 5). In this module, residents discuss the characteristics of an effective lecture and methods for stimulating interest and maximizing the effect of the lecture on the learner. Next, each resident presents a mini-lecture, preferably one that might be given during work or chart rounds. After that lecture, the speaker is asked to assess his own performance. What were the key points? What evidence suggests that the learners understood these points? What was most effective about the lecture? What was least effective? From the peer group the lecturer then receives comments, reinforcing effective skills and suggesting alternatives for ineffective ones. The faculty members complete the feedback process by summarizing the suggestions offered and linking the skills of effective lecturing to the principles of learning discussed in the first module. The session ends with a brief explanation of the next assignment, leading a small-group discussion.

Module 3: Leading a Small-Group Discussion

Resident teachers often have difficulty differentiating lecture from discussion and tend to lecture even when asked to lead a discussion. The objectives for this module include distinguishing between the skills required in lecturing and those needed for leading a discussion, setting a teaching agenda for discussion, devising questions appropriate for this agenda, and demonstrating methods for facilitating group participation.

To begin the session, we review the components of an effective discussion, emphasizing particularly the various functions that can be served by questions. The group then evaluates examples of questions drawn from the work-rounds observations. Which would elicit discussion? Which could be used to check for comprehension and understanding? Which would be appropriate for stimulating problem-solving?

Often raised for discussion by the residents is their own anxiety about leading a discussion of a topic without also being the "expert." The physician faculty members encourage the residents to consider the members of a discussion group as resources and the discussion as the beginning, not the endpoint, of learning. Exposing the unknown was presented as a means of promoting learning.

During the practice session, each resident facilitates a brief discussion, usually a case history revolving around a single clinical topic. The residents are encouraged to experiment with questions and examine the responses that different types of questions could elicit. After the discussion, the resident is asked to describe his discussion goals and to evaluate how well these goals were met. The group then talks over those features of the discussion that encouraged participation and comments on the types of questions used, often suggesting alternatives to ineffective questioning techniques.

In preparation for the next session, each resident is asked to select a case for presentation as if he were an intern with a new admission. This case will be presented to one of their peers who acts as a resident supervisor during a simulation of morning work rounds.

Module 4: One-to-One Teaching

The most realistic, yet complex, teaching activity addressed in the course, one-to-one teaching, obliges the supervising resident to respond to a clinical case. Teaching with a case combines components of role modeling, lecturing, discussion (especially the use of questions), and giving feedback—all without advance preparation. This module is intended to stimulate the formulation of a new model for impromptu teaching. Residents are challenged to consider how they might teach without foreknowledge of the particular case, handle the demands of patient care, and also address the educational needs of the learners. By the end of this module, residents should be able to explain several ways in which a case presentation can be used as a teaching activity and to identify different questioning techniques for fostering the development of clinical problem-solving skills.

In the introductory presentation, the faculty member asks the residents to consider the teaching goals that might be achieved through case presentations during work or teaching rounds: verifying skills in history-taking and physical examination, encouraging clinical decision-making, assisting in the setting of priorities for patient-care responsibilities, giving feedback on clinical performance and management decisions, and using disagreements and unanswered questions to stimulate learning.

During the simulation of work rounds, each resident is paired with an "intern" and charged with the task of teaching using the case presentation.The feedback that follows includes self-evaluation, "intern" evaluation, and comments from those observing the interaction.

Political Perspective

The history of the Clinical Teaching Skills Course shows how forces within an institution affect program initiation and continuation. The course was offered four times at Michael Reese Hospital and then discontinued because the four originators left for other institutions. The failure of the Department of Medicine to assign responsibility for the course to other faculty members, despite positive course evaluations by the house staff, is clear evidence of the importance of ensuring consistent departmental commitment.

Although the course was begun at the request of the Department of Medicine, no departmental leader participated in later course offerings. The importance of a central authority figure was realized when problems with scheduling, attendance, interruptions, and absences were encountered. We perceived these logistical problems as reducing the course's effectiveness.

To address these problems in planning later courses, we have required that certain conditions be met. These include (1) requiring attendance, (2) scheduling course time that does not conflict with other departmental programs, (3) ensuring that residents are relieved of their patient-care responsibilities during course time, (4) sending all information regarding the course directly from the chief resident or residency director's office, and (5) obtaining a commitment that the course is considered an important and integral part of the residency training program. Cooperative planning between departmental leaders and the course faculty members has led to fewer logistical problems in later offerings.

Analysis of why the course was not adopted into the residency program at Michael Reese Hospital also highlights the need to understand the climate in which a course is developed and implemented. The first step in this analysis is to determine institutional or departmental priorities and level of commitment to the course. Where does teaching fit into the department's priorities? How well is the concept "faculty development" understood? Who has recognized the existence of a problem that this course might address? Who has the authority to determine solutions? Who provides leadership and has responsibility for ensuring the success of the course? Is this person willing and able to participate in the course?

Currently, each request for the course triggers an analysis of the requesting department's political climate. Discussing the course "requirements" enables us to assess the departmental commitment as well as to establish the foundation for integrating the course into the residency program.

COURSE EVALUATION

A total of 175 residents participated in the Clinical Teaching Skills Course since the original pilot offering in August 1983. Although no course now exists at Michael Reese Hospital, the course is currently offered in six clinical departments at the Chicago College of Osteopathic Medicine.

For the first formal offering of the course at Michael Reese in December 1983, several evaluation methods were utilized. That first version relied more heavily on discussion than on practice and included only two practice-teaching sessions. To determine the quality and impact of this course, we developed three measures. First, participants completed a self-assessment questionnaire both before and after the course. The questionnaire asked residents to indicate the nature and quality of current teaching efforts and their perceived use of various teaching skills. Second, the participants completed a post-course satisfaction form that included an open-ended question asking for information on any changes in their teaching behavior as a result of the course. Finally, we observed the medical residents during work rounds both before and after the course.

The self-assessment of teaching skills indicated that at the end of the course all of the participants remained dissatisfied with the amount of teaching that they were doing on work rounds and wanted to do more. Now, however, they uniformly expressed an increased sense of confidence in their ability to teach. After the course, residents indicated that they were slightly better at asking problem-solving questions, generalizing from specific patient findings, pacing rounds for teaching, and leading the team. Four of the participants indicated that as a result of the course they were taking more time to ask and answer questions during work rounds.

When asked to evaluate the quality of the course, all of the participants rated the course as "excellent" or "good." All believed that the course content was "extremely useful" or "somewhat useful." According to the residents, the most useful aspects of the course were the practice sessions, the feedback received from peers, and the opportunity to observe the teaching styles of other residents. To improve the course, they suggested that more time be given for practice and peer critique by reducing the time devoted to discussion.

Postcourse observations were done on 12 of the 14 residents who had participated in the precourse observational study. Six of the 12 residents had completed the Clinical Teaching Skills Course 3 months earlier. The remaining six had not attended the course and served as the control group. Each resident was observed during one work-rounds session while reviewing an average of 10 patients. Results of the postcourse observations must be viewed with caution.First, the residents were assigned to different teams on different floors than they had been on during precourse observations. Second, 1 resident who had taken the course and 1 control were not included in the postcourse observations. Third, the residents were observed on only one occasion. Finally, increased attention to clinical teaching in the department may well have been created by the course and a concurrent study of departmental teaching rounds (Maxwell et al., 1983; Medio et al., 1984). Despite these possibly confounding variables, postcourse observations supported the residents' own assessments of the impact of the course on their behavior as teachers and provided important information for course revision.

Results of the postcourse observations showed that residents had changed in their use of questions. This change was of specific interest, given the focus of the teaching skills course. Residents who had taken the course showed a 14% increase in the frequency with which they asked members of the team to identify pertinent patient problems and a 15% increase in asking problem-solving questions. Although the control residents showed a similar increase in asking for patient problems, they showed a decrease (−5%) in the use of problem-solving questions.

As a result of resident feedback and the observational study, we revised the Clinical Teaching Skills Course in two major ways before offering it again. These changes are reflected in the description of course modules in the previous section. First, each module was revised to include role playing or practice teaching opportunities. Second, it had become apparent that residents valued the feedback provided by peers. The critical task for the faculty members was to develop techniques to facilitate peer critique while minimizing their own role in the feedback process. Table 13.2 lists the facilitator techniques developed for this purpose.

Subsequent course offerings have not included routine postcourse observations, except those done on an individual consultative basis to reinforce skills and facilitate adoption by the residents. Precourse observations have been continued for three reasons: (1) to familiarize the faculty with the specific teaching responsibilities of the residents who will be taking the course, (2) to gather examples of teaching for use during the course, and (3) to understand unique teaching constraints and team structure so that the course can be tailored for specific groups. As an example, surgical house staff have different opportunities to teach and have different demands on their time than do medical house staff. Identifying time to teach became a critical issue for the Clinical Teaching Skills Course for surgical residents.

Precourse and postcourse self-assessment and a postcourse satisfaction questionnaire have been collected for each course offering. Most residents have indicated that they are more confident in their teaching abilities after the course. Comments by residents indicated that their at-

TABLE 13.2 Facilitator Techniques for the Peer-Critique Session

1. Focus attention on teaching behaviors
2. Begin by asking the resident teacher for self-evaluation
3. Encourage balanced comments on effective and ineffective aspects of performance
4. Ask resident learners to provide feedback on teaching skills and learning outcomes
5. Reinforce the use of focused, descriptive feedback
6. Promote discussion of alternatives to ineffective aspects of performance
7. Summarize strengths, problems, and suggestions made by the group
8. Add faculty feedback at the end to avoid preempting peer and self-evaluation

titudes toward teaching had changed and they were using specific teaching skills:

> "You don't have to know vast details about a subject in order to teach."
> "I now consider five-minute talks more valuable."
> "I try to stimulate interest and to ask challenging questions without clear answers."
> "I have others identify problems, formulate plans, and discuss their knowledge."
> "More pausing for feedback."
> "More questioning and more structuring of time."
> "Frequently find myself falling back to the 'bad habit' of just directing and doing, instead of asking and explaining, especially when pressed for time, and now I am aware of it!"

All of the residents who have taken the course have rated it "excellent" or "good" and the content "extremely useful" or "useful." Residents have continually noted the use of active participation as a strength of the course.

Ongoing course evaluations indicate that the residents believe that they have learned more through the self-discovery generated during the practice teaching and peer-critique sessions than from the more didactic portions of the course. As a result of this perception, the role of the faculty in the course has evolved from instructor to that of facilitator. Of particular importance has been the ability of the faculty members to provide a safe environment in which new skills can be practiced, to evoke self-evaluation, and to guide the residents in offering specific, descriptive feedback to one another.

By virtue of its flexible design, the Clinical Teaching Skills Course continues to be responsive to the needs of residents from different departments and different institutions. The modular format, use of precourse observations to ensure a specific tailoring of emphasis, and postcourse revisions based on resident feedback provide the mechanisms for ensuring that the course can serve the needs of a diverse group of learners.

CHAPTER 14

Resident Teaching: A Critical Review and Future Projections

JANINE C. EDWARDS
WARREN C. PLAUCHÉ
ROBERT L. MARIER

RESIDENT TEACHING IN THE FUTURE

For residents, teaching occupies a priority lower than patient care and their own medical training. For faculty also, teaching ranks lower than patient care and research. This order of priority must be recognized. Teaching improvement programs must fit into the structures and routines of residency programs and clinical settings; otherwise, they will be ignored.

To develop the role of residents as teachers, it will be important to gain approval from residency-accrediting agencies for teaching skills to be a component of clinical competence. In this way, teaching may be allowed to take its rightful, albeit third, place in residency training. Then in time, the concept of teaching as an integral part of the residency experience may be accepted by all those persons involved in training students and residents, and may be incorporated into the routine evaluations of residents' performance.

The structure of residency programs is changing because of economic conditions in the health care field. Exactly how these changes will impact on residency training in the future is unclear as yet. The clinical training of medical students, however, is so intricately tied to the patient-care system that students will almost certainly continue to be supervised, at least in part, by residents. Furthermore, in many schools faculty are being encouraged to expand their clinical practice to provide financial support for themselves and the institution. This trend will allow faculty less time to teach. The traditional teaching role of residents may take on added importance in the future.

Research Needed

The studies described by Weinholtz (Chapter 8 in this volume) and by other reports are needed to build a sound base of information about current teaching responsibilities and the status quo of residents' skills. Observations of several teams' work rounds would provide a broad, horizontal view of one type of teaching activity. Only two such studies have been reported (Tremonti and Biddle, 1982; Wilkerson et al., 1986). In addition to the direct observation of residents on work rounds as recommended by Weinholtz, we think that a multisite series of case studies would contribute greatly to this field. Case studies could lead to a vertical, in-depth analysis of the teaching of residents as they develop through their years of medical training. The residents for case studies could be selected to represent each category of the taxonomy explained in the Preface: the intuitive teachers, the willing teachers who need training, and the residents unmotivated to teach. Comprehensive observational studies of residents' activities are needed to generate a total concept of all the teaching opportunities that residents have and the teaching methods residents actually use. Work rounds may not be the most productive teaching opportunity for residents. Indeed, our observations indicate that the most creative teaching activities can occur during unscheduled ward work.

Our observations have showed the importance of residents' management techniques, an idea also pointed out by Weinholtz (Chapter 8, p. 131) and by Meleca and Pearsol (Chapter 11, p. 193). If the clinical team is not managed efficiently, time and energy for teaching are frittered away. Studies of various strategies used to manage ward teams efficiently are needed.

Data accumulated from basic descriptive research could supply answers to such research questions as (1) Why do some residents teach while others do not? (2) How can residents be motivated to teach? (3) What types of learning can residents teach? (4) Who benefits best from teaching skills programs? (5) What teaching techniques work best for residents?

The case studies in this book show that many assumptions have been made in response to the research questions raised above, and that the designs for improvement programs rest on those assumptions. Programs would doubtless be more effective and longer lasting if concrete answers to these questions were known. A body of knowledge about the reality of resident teaching must be built. Empirical facts must be observed, compared across settings, and accumulated to give a comprehensive, accurate picture of resident teaching.

The case studies in Part III of this volume also show that most improvement program developers are educators, although clinicians are team members. During the planning stage, the educators observed resident and attending physician teaching. Although these observations served to orient them to the life and duties of residents and provided some specific material for the improvement programs they developed, much more information could be gained from formal observational studies.

Why has so little attention been given previously to formal observational studies? Until recently, most educational researchers were not trained in descriptive or qualitative research methods. Methods of case study and ethnography have been the traditional province of sociologists and anthropologists. Bosk (1979), for example, who described the methods used to control errors among surgery residents, was a sociologist. Educational researchers have been trained in the past in quantitative experimental research methods, including psychometrics. Currently there is much interest among educators in descriptive research. If this interest continues, descriptions of the clinical teaching of residents may emerge.

Time for Teaching

Finding time to teach is a problem for residents. Heavy demands of patient care and their own structured educational activities (conferences, grand rounds, and the like) leave little time and energy for anything else. Yet the teaching responsibility is a day-to-day reality. Residents must develop awareness of opportunities to teach as they work with patients. In this way, their teaching proceeds simultaneously with their work and requires little additional time.

Another problem is finding time for a teaching improvement program. The case studies illustrate two ways of finding time: (1) taking residents out of the work context for a short course and (2) providing several 1- or 2-hour sessions woven into residency routines. Both types of instruction have proved feasible, and, indeed, a combination of both types seems necessary to increase skill. A short course could be given annually to heighten awareness and understanding of teaching principles. Short sessions three or four times a year that can fit into a regular schedule of case conferences, ethics conferences, or grand rounds are feasible. Spacing instruction over time reinforces its effectiveness (Stritter 1983, p. 30). For some individuals a more intensive method, such as videotaping and critiquing, may be necessary. The optimum time for delivering these types of instruction seems to be from the middle of the first year through the middle of the second year. New interns have so many adjustment problems to deal with early in their first year that further demands seem almost sadistic. Stritter describes the stresses of the internship year and the intellectual maturing during later years. Additionally, interns usually are not given the actual responsibility for student teaching, or evaluation. To reap the maximum benefits of enhanced teaching, however, instruction must begin rather early in the residency program and capitalize on the steep learning curve of clinical competence. The last year of residency is too late; at that time teaching may be perceived as desirable only by those who are planning careers in academia.

Results of Teaching Improvement Programs

The case studies in this book are concrete evidence that interest in the teaching role of residents is increasing and that many medical schools are developing improvement programs. Furthermore, evaluation results from several sources show that residents' teaching skills can be improved (Table 14.1). In Chapter 9, Edwards et al. (p. 173) found that residents who received instruction were scored higher by trained raters of videotapes on a number of specific clinical teaching skills than were control residents. Jewett et al. (1982) found that residents who received instruction in teaching expressed more confidence in their teaching and considered this responsibility a higher priority than they did before the instruction. Ratings of students, peers, and faculty of these residents were consistently higher than those of residents who had not received instruction. Lawson and Harvill (1980) showed that residents scored higher on videotape ratings after instruction than they did before instruction, and that residents reported more positive attitudes about teaching after instruction than before. In Chapter 13, Medio et al. (pp. 225–226) observed residents several months after they received instruction and noted some improvement in the asking of problem-solving questions. All teaching improvement programs that evaluated effectiveness have showed positive results.

TABLE 14.1 Evaluation Results of Teaching Improvement Programs for Residents

Programs	Design	Results
Edwards et al. Chapter 9	Experimental/control groups Medicine, Family Medicine, Ob/Gyn	Videotape ratings: experimental > control
Edwards et al. Chapter 9	Experimental/control groups (HOI) All specialties	1. Post > pre self-ratings 2. Students rated experimental HOIs > control HOIs
Jewett et al. 1982	Experimental/control groups (HOIs, IIs IIIs) Pediatrics	1. Self-report: experimental > controls on confidence in teaching 2. Ratings by students, faculty, peers: experimental > control 3. Confidence in teaching positively correlated with need for warmth and approval from others
Lawson and Harvill (1980)	One group, pre- and posttest Family Medicine and Medicine	1) Videotaped ratings: post > pre 2) Attitudes self-report: Post- more positive than pre-
Medio et al. Chapter 13	Experimental/control groups Medicine	Experimental group 15% increase and control group 5% decrease in problem-solving questions

We should point out that Irby's chapter on evaluation differs from the evaluation of program effectiveness presented in the case studies (Chapters 10 and 11). In those case study chapters, the focus is on determining how effectively the program improved residents' teaching. In education, this is termed evaluation research. Once the effectiveness of specific educational methods has been substantiated, such evaluation will not be necessary for every program.

Use of Theories in Practical Ways

Many theoretical perspectives from medicine, education, psychology, and sociology can enrich clinical teachers' experience. A better understanding of both processes might exist today had a rich array of theories from various fields been related to clinical learning and teaching in the past. The paucity of perspectives within which clinical education has been studied has severely limited understanding of its complexity. Skeff, in Chapter 6, summarizes various theories that can be useful in developing teaching improvement programs. The theories are organized into two categories, those dealing with attitudes and those concerning knowledge and skills.

Although the two categories are of equal importance, in medicine less attention is likely to be given to attitudes than to cognition. For this reason, we emphasize the relevance of motivating residents to participate in teaching improvement programs. Need theory, motive-acquisition theory, self-efficiency theory, and adult-learning theory can stimulate ideas about approaches to resident teaching improvement programs that will avoid pitfalls and build in success.

Other applications of various theories help illustrate the importance of thinking explicitly about these perspectives. At Louisiana State University, we considered role modeling or social-learning theory important. Therefore, clinical faculty members were involved from the beginning in planning and in teaching the program because they are role models for residents. Furthermore, senior residents of outstanding ability from the various departments were involved because they too are role models for their peers.

Cognitive psychology has potential for understanding problem-solving. Chapters 1 and 4 incorporate cognitive psychology to explain the dual processes of learning and teaching. Artificial intelligence (AI), the nexus of many disciplines, holds the potential for modeling human thought processes on computers. Future advances in these fields should yield information about how to teach clinical reasoning.

A good theory is practical. Considering the implications of the theories in Chapter 6 for teaching improvement programs can ensure success.

Methods for Improving Teaching

Skeff and his associates (Chapter 6) have reviewed studies using various methods for improving teaching: those studies are summarized in Table 14.2. They conclude that multicomponent methods—seminars and workshops—show most evidence of effectiveness, although the

TABLE 14.2 Methods for Improving Teaching

Method	Studies	Effectiveness
Feedback from student ratings	Rotem and Glasman (1979) Rous et al. (1972) Stillman et al. (1983) Skeff (1983)	Not consistently effective
Feedback with self-assessment, consultation, or booklets	Pambookian (1976) Centra (1973) Aleamoni (1978) McKeachie (1979) Cohen and Herr (1982)	More effective than feedback alone
Peer review	Centra (1975) Sweeney and Grasha (1978) Sell (1986) Adams et al. (1974) Skeff (1981) Medio et al. (1987)	Somewhat effective; may be more useful for residents than faculty
Consultation with a professional educator	Foley et al. (1976) Irby et al. (1976) Partridge et al. (1980) Wergin et al. (1976)	Effective
Videotape review	Kagan (1975) Gliesman and Pugh (1978a; 1978b) Allen and Ryan (1969) Bazuin and Yonke (1978) Cassie et al. (1977) Foley et al. (1976) Mahler and Benor (1984) Sheets and Henry (1984) Skeff et al. (1983) Skeff et al. (1982) Lawson and Harvill (1980) Meleca and Schimpf-hauser (1976) Edwards et al. (1987) Jewett et al. (1982)	Effective
Self-evaluation	Carroll (1981) Seldin (1980)	Effectiveness not known

TABLE 14.2 (*Continued*)

Method	Studies	Effectiveness
Concept-based training	Gliessman and Pugh (1984) Skeff et al. (1986)	Effective
Multicomponent methods: seminars and workshops	Mahler and Benor (1984) Skeff et al. (1986) Lawson and Harvill (1980) Jewett et al. (1982) Edwards et al. (1987) Medio et al. (1987)	Effective

relative contribution of each component has not been identified. Other effective methods include consultation with a professional educator, videotape review, and concept-based training. Peer review may be more useful for residents than it has been for faculty, because residents work closely together and learn from each other. Feedback from student ratings, if combined with other methods, may be useful.

Content for Teaching Improvement Programs

Content for teaching improvement programs is generally not available. Most programs have had to develop their own. There is no well-developed, standardized curriculum. A few articles in medical and medical education journals as well as several chapters in this book describe teaching techniques. A body of research on medical problem-solving and decision analysis exists. Beyond that, one must look at educational and psychological research and theory and attempt to apply it in clinical settings. A curriculum of clinical teaching skills and instructional materials are needed. In addition, attending physicians need instruments for evaluating resident teaching skills. Observations of clinical teaching and the assessment of learning outcomes are needed to develop these materials.

Instructors for Teaching Improvement Programs

The planning phase of a new program is critical. Regardless of where the idea begins, multiple levels of faculty and administrators must be involved. Teaching enhancement projects are included in the mission of almost all medical schools, but these must be actively supported at the highest levels of administration if they are to succeed. The residency director is the key figure in developing a successful teaching program for residents. If the director supports the program, it is likely to be successful. On the other hand, if he ignores or opposes it, the program probably will not survive for long. Three of the case studies in this volume give negative and positive examples of this observation (Chapters 9, 10, and 13). Furthermore, specific and active involvement of the director in the planning and teaching of the program will undoubtedly assure its success. The department head's support is also important because that person influences all units within the department.

We think the best approach today to developing a program of teaching improvement is to draw on the experience and opinions of excellent clinical teachers, faculty and residents. Those who teach well in clinical settings can provide essential information about it. Physicians who also have degrees in education or extensive educational knowledge and experience are ideal leaders for teaching improvement programs. Educators and psychologists can contribute information from their disciplines. A team of physicians and educators is certainly workable, and in most medical settings such collaboration is probably the most feasible approach. All of the case studies in this book are examples of such collaboration. It should be noted, however, that the degree of collaboration varied among teams.

Senior residents are the third essential element of the team. These residents must be enthusiastic volunteers, because their roles will require valuable time. They must have seniority in their programs in order to back their opinions with experience. Senior residents know the timing of all program activities and can spot schedule conflicts. They command the respect of those below them and are able to motivate junior residents to attend teaching skills programs sessions despite other demands on their time. Older clinicians, respected though they may be, have not been "on the wards" as the residents are, day in and day out. Senior residents know what types of teaching are going on, and they can recognize what opportunities could be better used. The immediacy of their ward experiences cannot be substituted for by anyone else.

During the actual teaching of the program, the clinicians on the team have several roles. They are important role models. They also act as content experts, and they can field the medical questions that arise.

One must be aware that an educator acting alone has a problem establishing credibility with physician audiences. Physicians in training most readily accept the opinions of other physicians, principally their own residency director. Each educator must win the respect of at least a few clinicians in his setting before he can work effectively. The educator may have to go through informal rites of passage to demonstrate his intelligence, professional competence, leadership, ability to work, and his willingness to contribute whatever he can to the medical setting. Clinicians can enhance the credibility of educators by showing respect for them as colleagues.

Ideally, as we have described, a teaching improvement program for residents has some faculty physicians actively involved in planning and teaching. Residents want to know that faculty members are involved in development programs for their own improvement. They will resent efforts to improve their teaching if faculty are not making equal efforts. Clinical education has shared responsibilities, as does patient care. A teaching improvement program could begin with either faculty or residents, but it inevitably must include both groups.

The Future

What does the future hold for resident teaching? Health care delivery systems are already increasingly oriented toward prevention of disease, cost containment, and outpatient settings. Teaching skills will augment residents' ability to function in these areas. Developing programs for teaching skills in these settings will be challenging.

Biomedical and computer technology are forging ahead rapidly. These advances create new knowledge and skills that physicians must continue to learn throughout their careers. At the same time, computer technology is opening up new opportunities for teaching and avenues for communicating.

CONCLUSIONS

Teaching skills are an important component of professional competence. Indeed, the word *doctor* means teacher. Physicians in training should have the privilege to learn to teach (that is, to cultivate intellectual growth), as well as to cultivate the physical health of persons associated with them. Teaching skills should be included in residency curriculum and evaluation systems. Further work is needed to develop teaching skills programs and materials.

References

Adams, W.R., Ham, T.H., Mawardi, B.H., Scali, H.A., and Weisman, R. 1964. A Naturalistic Study of Teaching in a Clinical Clerkship. *Journal of Medical Education, 39*: 164–174.

Adams, W.R., Ham, T.H., Mawardi, B.H., Scali, H.A., and Weisman, R. 1974. Research in Self-Education for Clinical Teachers. *Journal of Medical Education, 49*: 1166–73.

Aleamoni, L.M. 1978. The Usefulness of Student Evaluations in Improving College Teaching. *Instructional Science, 7*: 95–105.

Aleamoni, L. 1981. Student Ratings of Instruction. In *Handbook of Teacher Evaluation,* edited by J. Millman. London: Sage.

Aleamoni, L.M. and Hexner, P.Z. 1980. A Review of the Research on Student Evaluation and Report on the Effect of Different Sets of Instructions on Student Course and Instructor Evaluation. *Instructional Science 9:*67–84.

Allen, D.W., and Ryan, K. 1969. *Microteaching*. Reading, MA: Addison-Wesley.

Alpert, J.J., Yongerman, J., Breslow, J. and Kosa, J. 1973. Learning Experiences During the Internship Year: An Exploratory Study of Pediatric Graduate Education. *Pediatrics 51:*199–205.

American Board of Internal Medicine. 1979. Clinical Competence in Internal Medicine. *Annals of Internal Medicine, 90*: 402–410.

American Medical Association. 1986. *1986–1987 Director of Residency Training Programs*. Accredited by the Accreditation Council for Graduate Medical Education. Chicago.

Anderson, J.R. 1985. *Cognitive Psychology and Its Implications*. 2d ed. New York: W.H. Freeman.

Anderson, W.A., Bridgham, R.G., Alquire, P.C., and Mayle, J.E. 1984. Improving Medical Students' Clinical Case Presentation Skills. Paper presented at the Annual Meeting of the American Educational Research Association, New Orleans, LA.

Ashton, P. 1984. Teacher Efficiency: A Paradigm for Effective Teacher Education. *Journal of Teacher Education, 35*(5): 28–32.

Association of American Medical Colleges. 1976. *Clinical Supervision: A Written Simulation*.

Association of American Medical Colleges. 1984. Physicians for the twenty-first century. *Journal of Medical Education 59*:3–31.

Ausubel, D.P. 1968. *Educational Psychology: A Cognitive View*. New York: Holt, Rinehart & Winston.

Bandura, A. 1977. Self-Efficiacy: Toward a Unifying Theory of Behavioral Change, *Psychological Review, 84*: 191–215.

Barondess, J.A. 1985. Cushing and Osler—The Evaluation of a Friendship. *Transactions and Studies of the College of Physicians of Philadelphia, 7*: 79–112.

Barrett, J.A. 1984. A "Subskills" Method for Teaching Surgical Skills. *Focus on Surgical Education (ASE) Newsletter,* Vol. 1, No.3, summer issue.

Barrow, M.V. 1966. Medical Student Opinions of the House Officer as a Medical Educator. *Journal of Medical Education, 41*: 807–810.

Barrows, H.S. 1983. Problem-Based, Self-Directed Learning. *Journal of American Medical Association, 250*: 3077–380.

Barrows, H., and Tamblyn, R.M. 1980. *Problem Based Learning: An Approach to Medical Education*. New York: Springer Publishing Company.

Bates, J.A. 1979. Extrinsic Reward and Intrinsic Motivation: A Review with Implications for the Classroom. *Review of Educational Research, 49*(4): 557–576.

Bazuin, C.H., and Yonke, A.M. 1978. Improvement of Teaching Skills in a Clinical Setting. *Journal of Medical Education, 5*: 377–382.

Bean, W. B. 1985. Osler's Clinical Teaching. In *The Persisting Osler,* edited by J.A. Barondess, J. P. McGovern, and C. G. Roland, pp. 91–95. Baltimore: University Park Press.

Bell, R.M. 1984. Thoughts on Teaching Surgical Skills. *Focus on Surgical Education (ASE) Newsletter*. Vol. 1, No. 3, summer issue.

Berner, E. 1984. Paradigms and Problem-Solving: A Literature Review. *Journal of Medical Education, 59*: 625–633.

Biehler, R.F. 1978. *Psychology Applied to Teaching*. 3rd ed. New York: Houghton Mifflin Company.

Bland, C.J. 1980. *Faculty Development Through Workshops*. Springfield, IL: Charles C. Thomas.

Bligh, D. 1972. *What's the Use of Lectures*? New York: Penguin Books.

Bloom, B.S. et al, 1956a. *Taxonomy of Educational Objectives: Handbook I. Cognitive Domain*. New York: McKay.

Bloom, B.S. 1956b. *Taxonomy of Educational Objectives: The Classification of Educational Goals*. New York: Longmans Green.

Bobrow, S.A., and Bower, G.H. 1969. Comprehension and Recall of Sentences. *Journal of Experimental Psychology, 80*: 455–61.

Bosk, C.L. 1979. *Forgive and Remember: Managing Medical Failure*. Chicago: University of Chicago Press.

Bower, G.H., and Hilgard, E.R. 1981. *Theories of Learning*. Englewood Cliffs, NJ: Prentice-Hall.

Bronowski, J. 1978. *The Visionary Eye: Essays in the Arts, Literature, and Science*. Cambridge, MA: The MIT Press.

Brown, R.S. 1970. House Staff Attitudes Toward Teaching. *Journal of Medical Education, 45*: 156–159.

Brown, R., and Herrnstein, R.J. 1975. *Psychology*. Boston: Little, Brown.

Brown, T. R. 1920. Osler and the Student. In *Sir William Osler, Bart., Brief Tributes to His Personality, Influence, and Public Service*. Baltimore: Johns Hopkins University Press.

Bruner, J.S. 1966. *Toward a Theory of Instruction*. Cambridge, MA: Harvard University Press.

Brusling, C. 1974. *Microteaching—A Concept in Development*. Stockholm, Sweden: Almqvist and Wiksell International.

Bucher, R., and Snelling, J.G. 1977. *Becoming Professional*. Beverly Hills, CA: Sage Publications.

Bughman, E. 1973. Lecture Method of Instruction. In *Development of Educational Programs for the Health Professions*. Geneva: World Health Organization.

Camac, C.N.B. 1906. *Counsels and Ideals—from the Writings of William Osler*. Boston: Houghton Mifflin.

Cantrell, T. 1973. How do Medical-School Staff Learn to Teach? *Lancet, 2*: 724–727.

Carroll, J.G. 1981. Faculty Self-Evaluation. In J. Millman *Handbook of Teacher Evaluation,* edited by J. Millman, pp. 180–200 Beverly Hills, CA: Sage Publications.

Carroll, L. 1866. *Alice's Adventures in Wonderland*. London: Macmillan.

Cassie, J.M., Collins, G.F., and Daggett, C.J. 1977. The Use of Videotapes to Improve Clinical Teaching. *Journal of Medical Education, 52*(4): 353–354.

Centra, J. 1973. Self-ratings of college teachers: A comparison with student ratings. *Journal of Educational Measurement, 10*(4): 287–295.

Centra, J. 1975. Colleagues as Raters of Classroom Instruction. *Journal of Higher Education, 46*: 327–337.

Centra, J. 1976. *Faculty Development Practices in U.S. Colleges and Universities,* Princeton, NJ: Educational Testing Service.

Champagne, A.B., Gunstone, R.F., and Klopter, L.E. 1985. "Effecting Changes in Cognitive Structure Among Physics Students." In *Cognitive Structure and Conceptual Change,* edited by L.T.H. West and L.A. Pines, pp. 168–187. Orlando, FL: Academic Press.

Change Magazine. 1978. *Guide to Effective Teaching.*

Chi, M.T.H. Feltovich, P.J., and Glaser, R. 1981. Categorization and Representation of Physics Problems by Experts and Novices. *Cognitive Sciences, 5*: 151–152.

Clancey, W.J., Shortliffe, E.H., and Buchanan, B.G. 1984. Intelligent Computer-Aided Instruction for Medical Diagnosis. In *Readings in Medical Artifical Intelligence: The First Decade,* edited by W.J. Clancey and E.H. Shortliffe. Menlo Park, CA: Addison-Wesley.

Cohen, M.W. 1983. Using Motivation Theory as a Framework for Teacher Education. *Journal of Teacher Education, 34*(3), 10–13.

Cohen, P.A., and Herr, G. 1982. Using an Interactive Feedback Procedure to Improve College Teaching. *Teaching of Psychology, 9*(3): 138–140.

Collins, A., and Stevens, A.L. 1982. "Goals and Strategies of Inquiry Teachers."

In *Advances in Instructional Psychology, Volume II,* edited by R. Glaser, pp. 65–119. Hillsdale, NJ: Erlbaum.

Costin, G., Greenough, W.T., and Menges, R.J. 1971. Student Ratings of College Teaching: Reliability, Validity, and Usefulness. *Review of Educational Research, 41:* 511–535.

Cox, K.R., and Evan, C.E. 1982. *The Medical Teacher.* New York: Churchill Livingstone.

Cushing, H. 1940. *The Life of Sir William Osler.* 2 vols. New York: Oxford University Press.

Daggett, C.J. 1977. A Study to Determine the Role of Attending Physicians in Clinical Training of Medical Students and Resident Physicians. Doctoral dissertation. Amherst: University of Massachusetts.

Daggett, C.J., Cassie, J.M., and Collins, G.F. 1979. Research on Clinical Teaching, *Review of Educational Research, 49*:151–169.

Davis, R., and Alexander, L.T. 1977. *The Lecture Method.* East Lansing: Michigan State University.

Davison, W.C. 1973. Osler's Opposition to Whole-Time Clinical Professors. In *Humanism in Medicine,* edited by J. P. McGovern and C. R. Burns, pp. 30–33. Springfield, IL: Charles C. Thomas.

deCharms, R. 1976. *Enhancing Motivation: Change in the Classroom.* New York: Irvington.

Deci, E.L., and Ryan, R.M. 1982. Intrinsic Motivation to Teach: Possibilities and Obstacles in our Colleges and Universities. In *New Directions for Teaching and Learning: Motivating Professors to Teach Effectively,* edited by J.L. Bess. No. 10. San Francisco: Jossey-Bass.

Denzin, N.K. 1978. *The Research Act.* New York: McGraw-Hill.

Dewey, J. 1970. What Psychology Can Do For the Teacher. in *John Dewey on Education: Selected Writings,* edited by R. Archasmbault. New York: Associated Press.

Dutton, M.D., Seaman, D.F., and Ulmer, C. 1972. *Understanding Group Dynamics in Adult Education.* Englewood Cliffs, NJ: Prentice-Hall.

Edwards, J.C., Kissling, G.E., Plauché, W.C., and Marier, R.L. 1986. Long-Term Evaluation of Training Residents in Clinical Teaching Skills. *Journal of Medical Education, 61:* 967–970.

Edwards, J.C., Marier, R.L., and Kissling, G.E. 1985. Improving Clinical Teaching for Residents: Workshops and Seminars. *Professions Education Researcher Notes,* 7(2): 3–4.

Elstein, A.S., Shulman, L.S., and Sprafka, S.A. 1978. *Medical Problem Solving: An Analysis of Clinical Reasoning.* Boston: Harvard University Press.

Ende, J. 1983. Feedback in Clinical Medical Education. *Journal of American Medical Association, 250*: 777–781.

Engel, G.L. 1971. The Deficiencies of the Case Presentation as a Method of Clinical Teaching. *New England Journal of Medicine, 284*: 20–24.

Engel, G.L. 1965. "Clinical Observation: The Neglected Basic Method of Medicine." *Journal of the American Medical Association, 192*: 149–160.

Eraker, S.A., Kirschl, J.P., and Becker, M.H. 1984. Understanding and Improving Patient Compliance. *Annals Internal Medicine, 100*: 258–268.

Ericksen, S. 1980. "The Motivation to Remember". *Memo to the Faculty.* No. 67.

Ann Arbor: Center for Research on Learning and Teaching, University of Michigan.

Erickson, G.R., and Erickson, B.L. 1979. Improving College Teaching. *Journal of Higher Education, 50*(5): 670–683.

Farnham-Diggory, S. 1972. *Cognitive Processes in Education: A Psychological Preparation for Teaching and Curriculum Development.* New York: Harper & Row.

Feldman, D.H. 1980. *Beyond Universals in Cognitive Development.* Norwood, New Jersey: Ablex Publishing Co.

Feldman, I. 1976. The Superior College Teacher from the Student's View. *Research Higher Education, 5*: 243–288.

Feltovich, P.J. 1981. *Knowledge Based Components of Expertise in Medical Diagnosis.* Technical Report No. PDS-2. Pittsburgh: University of Pittsburgh, Learning Research and Development Center.

Feltovich, P.J., Johnson, P.E., Moller, J.H., and Swanson, D.B. 1984. "LCS: The Role and Development of Medical Knowledge in Diagnostic Expertise." In *Readings in Artificial Intelligence in Medicine: The First Decade,* edited by W.J. Clancey and E.H. Shortliffe, pp. 275–319. Reading, MA: Addison-Wesley.

Festinger, L. 1957. *A Theory of Cognitive Dissonance.* New York: Harper & Row.

Fidler, D.L., and Alexander, S. 1979. *G. Patton, M.D.* [videotape]. Chapel Hill, NC: Health Sciences Consortium.

Fitts, P.M. 1962. Factors in Complex Skill Training. In *Training Research* and *Evaluation,* edited by R. Glaser. New York: Wiley.

Flanders, N. 1974. Interaction Analysis: A Technique for Quantifying Teacher Influence. In Clarizio, H. et al. *Contemporary Issues in Educational Psychology.* 2d Edition, Boston: Allyn and Bacon.

Foley, R.P., and Smilansky, J. 1979. Teacher–Student Interaction in a Medical Clerkship. *Journal of Medical Education. 54*: 622–626.

Foley, R.P., and Smilansky, J. 1980. *Teaching Techniques: A Handbook for Health Professionals.* New York: McGraw-Hill.

Foley, R.P., Smilansky, J., Bughman, E., and Sajid, A. 1976. A Departmental Approach for Improving Lecture Skill of Medical Teachers. *Journal of Medical Education, 10*: 369–373.

Fuller, F.F., and Manning, B.A. 1973. Self-Confrontation Reviewed: A Conceptualization for Video Playback in Teacher Education. *Review of Educational Research, 43*: 469–528.

Frost, H.G. 1967. Observations on a great occasion. *Adult Education, 37*: 282.

Gaff, J.G. 1976. Overcoming Faculty Resistance. *New Directions for Higher Education, 4*: 43–57.

Gage, N.L. 1984. Hard Gains in the Soft Sciences. Bloomington, IN: *Phi Delta Kappa, 4.*

Gagné, E.D. 1985. *The Cognitive Psychology of School Learning.* Boston: Little, Brown.

Gagné, R.M. 1978. *The Conditions of Learning* (3rd ed.). New York: Holt, Rinehart & Winston.

Gagné, R.M., and Briggs, L.J. 1974. *Principles of Instructional Design*, New York: Holt, Rinehart & Winston.

Gardner, A. D. 1969. Some Recollections of Sir William Osler at Oxford. *Journal of the American Medical Association 210*: 2765–2766.

Giles, R.M., Johnson, M.R., Knight, K.E., Zammett, S., and Weinman, J. 1982. Recall of Lecture Information: A Question of What, When, and Where. *Medical Education, 16*: 264–268.

Glaser, R. 1984. Education and Thinking: The Role of Knowledge. *American Psychology, 39*: 93–104.

Gliessman, D.H., and Pugh, R.C. 1978a. Research on the Rationale, Design and Effectiveness of Protocol Materials. *Journal of Teacher Education, 29*(6): 87–91.

Gliessman, D.H., and Pugh, R.C. 1978b. Acquiring Teacher Behavior Concepts Through the Use of High Structure and Low Structure Protocol films. *Journal of Educational Psychology, 70*: 779–787.

Gliessman, D.H., and Pugh, R.C. 1984. Conceptual Variables in Teacher Training, *Journal of Education for Teaching, 10*(3): 195–208.

Graesser, A.C., and Black, J.B. (Eds.). 1985. *The Psychology of Questions*. Hillsdale, NJ: Erlbaum.

Greenberg, L.W., Goldberg, R.M. and Jewett, L.S. 1984. Teaching in the Clinical Settings: Factors Influencing Resident's Perceptions, Confidence and Behavior. *Medical Education 18:* 360–365.

Greenberg, L.W. and Jewett, L.S. 1983. Student Learning in a Pediatric Clerkship. *Journal of Medical Education 58:* 484–486.

Havinghurst, R.J. 1972. *Developmental Tasks and Education*. New York: McKay.

Higbee, K.L. 1977. *Your Memory: How It Works and How to Improve It*. Englewood Cliffs, NJ: Prentice-Hall.

Highet, G. 1950. *The Art of Teaching*, pp. 231, 236, 245. New York: Knopf.

Hinz, C.F. 1966. Direct Observation as a Means of Teaching and Evaluating Clinical Skills. *Journal of Medical Education, 41*: 150–151.

Hoban, J.D., and Camp, M.G. 1980. *Materials Related to Teaching in Medical School: A Preliminary Report*. Winston-Salem, NC: Bowman Gray School of Medicine.

Holman, E. 1969. Sir William Osler. *Journal of the American Medical Association, 210*: 2223.

Houle, C. O. 1969. A Firstling of his Heart and Hand. *Perspectives in Biology and Medicine, 12*: 561–583.

Howard, R. P. 1983. *The Chief: Doctor William Osler*. Canton, MA: Science History Publications U.S.A.

Howe, M. 1977. *Adult Learning*. New York: Wiley.

Hyman, R.T. 1979. *Strategic Questioning*. Englewood Cliffs, NJ: Prentice-Hall.

Inglefinger, F. 1978. "The Graying of Grand Rounds." *The New England Journal of Medicine, 299*: 772.

Inglis, S.C., and Marazon, D.J. 1983. *Clinical Teaching Resources for Physicians*. Athens, OH: Ohio University College of Osteopathic Medicine.

Irby, D. 1978a. Clinical Teacher Effectiveness in Medicine. *Journal of Medical Education, 53*: 808–815.

Irby, D. 1978b. Clinical Faculty Development. In *Clinical Education for the Allied Health Professions,* edited by C.W. Ford, pp. 95–110. St. Louis: Mosby.

Irby, D., DeMers, J., Scher, M., and Matthews, D. 1976. A Model for the Improvement of Medical Faculty Lecturing. *Journal of Medical Education, 51*: 403–409.

Irby, D.M., and Rakestraw, P.G. 1981. Evaluating Clinical Teaching In Medicine. *Journal of Medical Education, 56*: 181–186.

Irby, D.M., Vontver, L.A. and Stenchever, M.A. 1982. Improving Teaching in a Multi-Site Clerkship: Faculty Development Workshops. *Journal of Reproductive Medicine 27:* 307–330.

Jason, H.R. 1962. A Study of Medical Teacher Practices. *Journal of Medical Education, 37*: 258–261.

Jewett, L.S., Grant, L.W., and Greenberg, R.M. 1983. Factors influencing teaching effectiveness. *American Journal of Diseases of Children, 137*: 544.

Jewett, L.S., Greenberg, R.M., Acord, A.L. and Greenberg, L.W. 1982a. Teaching Management Problems: Their Use in the Development of Faculty and Resident Treaching Skills. Innovations in Medical Education Exhibits. Group on Medical Education, Association of American Medical Colleges.

Jewett, L.S., Greenberg, L.W. and Goldberg, R.M. 1982b. Teaching Residents How to Teach: A One Year Study. *Journal of Medical Education, 57*: 361–366.

Kagan, N. 1975. *Interpersonal Process Recall: A Method of Influencing Human Interaction.* Maston, MI: Mason Media.

Kassirer, J.P. 1983. Iterative Hypothesis Testing: Let's Preach What We Practice. *New England Journal of Medicine, 309*: 921–925.

Kassirer, J.P., and Gorry, G.A. 1978. Clinical Problem Solving: A Behavioral Analysis. *Annals of Internal Medicine, 89*: 245–255.

Katona, G. 1940. *Organizing and Memorizing.* New York: Columbia Univeristy Press.

Kenny, Michael. 1982. *Presenting Yourself.* New York: Wiley.

Kestin, John. 1970. "Creativity in Teaching and Learning." *American Scientist, 53*: 250–257.

Klatzky, R.L. 1980. *Human Memory* 2d ed. New York: W.H. Freeman.

Knowles, M. 1978. *The Adult Learner: A Neglected Species.* Houston, TX: Gulf.

Knowles, M. 1970. *The Modern Practice of Adult Education.* New York: Associated Press.

Kohlberg, L. 1976. Moral Stages and Moralization: The Cognitive Developmental Approach. In *Moral Development and Behavior,* edited by T. Lickons. New York: Holt, Rinehart & Winston.

Kosslyn, S.M. 1980. *Image and Mind.* Cambridge, MA: Harvard University Press.

Kroenke, K. 1984. The Lecture: Where It Wavers. *The American Journal of Medicine, 77*: 393–396.

Lawson, B.K., and Harvill, L.M. 1980. The Evaluation of a Training Program for Improving Residents' Teaching Skills. *Journal of Medical Education, 55*: 1000–1005.

Lesgold, A.M., Rubinson, H. and Feltovich, P.J. In press. Expertise in a Complex Skill: Diagnosing X-ray Pictures.

Levinson-Rose, J. and Menges, R.J. 1981. Improving College Teaching: A Critical Review of Research. *Review of Educational Research, 51*: 403–434.

Linfors, E.W., and Neelon, F.A. 1980. The Case for Bedside Rounds. *New England Journal of Medicine 303*: 1230–1233.

Loevinger, J. 1976. *Ego development*. San Francisco: Jossey-Bass.

Lofland, J. 1971. *Analyzing social settings*. Belmont, CA: Wadsworth.

Lowman, Joseph. 1984. *Mastering the Techniques of Teaching*. San Francisco: Jossey-Bass.

Ludmerer, K.M. 1985. *Learning to Heal—the Development of American Medical Education*. New York: Basic Books.

Maddox, H., and Hoole, E. 1975. Performance Decrement in the Lecture. *Educational Review, 28*: 17–30.

Mager, R.F. 1972. *Goal Analysis*. Belmont, CA: Fearon Publishing.

Mahler, S., and Benor, D.E. 1984. Short and Long Term Effects of a Teacher-Training Workshop in Medical School. *Higher Education, 13*; 265–273.

Marsh, H.W. and Overall, J.U. 1979. Long-Term Stability of Student's Evaluations: A Note on Feldman's "Consistency and Variability among College Students in Rating Their Teachers and Courses." *Research on Higher Education 8*: 39–47.

Marx, M.H. and Bunch, M.E. 1977. *Fundamentals and Applications of Learning.* New York: Macmillan.

Maslow, A.H. 1954. *Motivation and Personality*. New York: Harper & Row.

Mattern, W.D., Weinholtz, D., and Friedman, C.P. 1983. The Attending Physician as Teacher. *New England Journal of Medicine, 308*: 1129–1132.

Maxwell, J.A., Cohen, R.M., and Reinhard, J.D. 1983. A Qualitative Study of Teaching Rounds in a Department of Medicine. *Proceedings of the Annual Conference on Research in Medical Education, 21*:192–197.

McCall, G.J., and Simmons J.L. 1969. *Issues In Participant Observation*. Reading, MA: Addison-Wesley.

McClelland, D.C. 1965. Toward a Theory of Motive Acquisition. *American Psychologist, 20*: 321–333.

McGovern, J.P. 1985. Wilbert C. Davison—Apostle of the Osler Tradition. In *The Persisting Osler,* edited by J.A. Barondess, J.P. McGovern, and C. G. Roland, pp. 265–276. Baltimore: University Park Press.

McGovern, J.P., and Roland, C.G. (Eds.). 1969. *William Osler—The Continuing Education,* pp. 53–57, 224. Springfield, IL: Charles C Thomas.

McGuire, C. 1984. Medical Problem-Solving: A Critique of the Literature. *Proceedings of the Twenty-third Annual Conference of Research in Medical Education, 23*: 1–13.

McKeachie, W. 1965. *Teaching Tips*. Lexington, MA: Heath.

McKeachie, W.J. 1979. Student Ratings of Faculty : A Reprise. *Academe, 65*: 384–397

McLeish, J. 1976. "The Lecture Method". In *The Psychology of Teaching Methods,* edited by N.L. Gage. Chicago: The University of Chicago Press.

McMaster University. 1981. Resident as Teacher. *Pedagogue, 10*: 1-3.

Medio, F.J., Wilkerson, L., Maxwell, J.A., Cohen, R.M., and Reinhard, J.D. 1984. Improving Teaching Rounds: Action Research in Medical Education. *Proceedings of the Annual Conference on Research in Medical Education, 23*: 283-288.

Meleca, C.B. and Schimpfhauser, F. 1976. A House Staff Training Program to Improve the Clinical Instructor. Paper presented to the Conference on Research in Medical Education, Washington, DC.

Mouw, D.R. 1981. "Using the Personal (Very Personal) Anecdote". *New Directions for Teaching and Learning, 7*: 27-30.

Napell, S.M. 1976. Six Common Non-facilitating Teaching Behaviors. *Contemporary Education, 47*(2).

National Medical Audiovisual Center. 1976. *Storyboarding/Visualizing Virtues.* [Videotape]. Atlanta, GA: Author

Neisser, U. 1967, *Cognitive Psychology.* New York: Appleton-Century-Crofts.

Norman D. 1982. *Learning and Memory.* New York: W.H. Freeman.

Norman, G.R., Tugwell, P., Feightner, J.W., Muzzin, L.G., and Jacoby, L.L. 1985. Knowledge and Clinical Problem-Solving. *Medical Education, 19*: 344-356.

Osler, W. 1892. *Principles and Practice of Medicine.* New York: Appleton and Company.

Osler, W. 1899. After twenty-five years. *Montreal Medical Journal, 28*: 823-833.

Osler, W. 1901. Books and Men. *Boston Medical and Surgical Journal, 144*: 60-61.

Osler, W. 1905. The Fixed Period. *Journal of American Medical Association, 44*:705-710.

Osler, W. 1907. The Reserves of Life. *St. Mary's Hospital Gazette, 13*: 95-98.

Osler, W. 1909. The Treatment of Disease. *Canada Lancet, 42*: 899-912.

Osler, W. 1911a. On the Hospital Unit in University Work. *Northumberland and Durham Medical Journal, 18*: 178-189.

Osler, W. 1911b. The Pathological Institute of a General Hospital. *Glasgow Medical Journal, 76*: 321-333.

Osler, W. 1945. *Aequanimitas with Other Addresses* 3rd ed. Philadelphia: Blakeston.

Osler, W. 1962. Letter to President Ira Remsen of Johns Hopkins, September 1, 1911. *Canadian Medical Association Journal, 87*: 762-765.

Osler, W. 1969. *A Way of Life—An Address Delivered to Yale Students, April 20, 1913.* Springfield, IL: Charles C. Thomas.

Pambookian, J.S. 1976. Discrepancy Between Instructor and Student Evaluations of Instruction: Effect on Instruction. *Instructional Science, 5*: 63-75.

Patridge, M.I., Harris, I.B., and Petzel, R.A. 1980. Implementation and Evaluation of a Faculty Development Program to Improve Clinical Teaching, *Journal of Medical Education, 55*: 711-713.

Pauker, S.G., and Kassirer, J.P. 1980. The Threshold Approach to Clinical Decision Making. *New England Journal of Medicine, 302*: 1109–1117.

Payson, H.E., and Barchas, J.D. 1965. A Time Study of Medical Teaching Rounds. *New England Journal of Medicine, 273*: 1468–1471.

Penner, J.G. 1984. *Why Many College Teachers Cannot Lecture.* Springfield, IL: Charles C. Thomas.

Perlberg, A. 1983. When Professors Confront Themselves: Towards a Theoretical Conceptualization of Video Self-Confrontation in Higher Education. *Higher Education, 12*: 633–663.

Perry, D.R., Challoner, D.R., and Oberst, R.J. 1981. Research Advances and Resource Constraints: Dilemmas Facing Medical Education. *New England Journal of Medicine, 305*: 320–324.

Perry, W.G.J. 1970. *Forms of Intellectual and Ethical Development in the College Years: A Scheme.* New York: Holt, Rinehart & Winston.

Petzel, R.A., Harris, I.B., and Masler, D.S. 1982. The Empirical Validation of Clinical Teaching Strategies. *Evaluation and the Health Professions, 5*: 499–508.

Piaget, J. 1963. *The Psychology of Intelligence.* Paterson, N.J.: Littlefield Adams.

Piaget, J. 1972. Intellectual Development from Adolescence to Adulthood. *Human Development, 15*: 1–12.

Popham, W.J. 1973. *The Uses of Instructional Objectives.* Belmont, CA: Feason Publications.

Posner, M.I., and Keele, S.W. 1973. Skill Learning, In *Second Handbook of Research on Teaching,* edited by R.M.W. Travers. Chicago: Rand McNally.

Prater, M., and Laputz, C. 1984. A Structured Approach to Clinical Skills Instruction. *Focus on Surgical Education (ASE) Newsletter,* Vol. 1, No.3., summer issue.

Pratt, J. H. 1949. *A Year with Osler—1896–1897.* Baltimore: The Johns Hopkins University Press.

Reichsman, F., Browning, F.E., and Hinshaw, J.R. 1964. Observations of Undergraduate Clinical Teaching in Action. *Journal of Medical Education, 39*: 147–153.

Reuler, J.B., Nardone, D.A., Elliot, D.L., and Girard, D.E. 1982. Education for Clinical Medicine: An Annotated Bibliography of Recent Literature. *Annals of Internal Medicine, 97*: 624–629.

Rezler, A.G. and French, R.M. 1975. Personality Types of Learning Preferences of Students in Six Allied Health Professions. *Journal of Allied Health 4*: 20–26.

Richardson, E. H. 1959. *A Doctor Remembers.* New York: Vantage Press.

Riegel, K.F. 1973. Dialectic Operations: The Final Period of Cognitive Development. *Human Development, 16*: 346–370.

Rogers, F. B. 1974. William Osler: Teacher. *Transactions and Studies of the College of Physicians of Philadelphia, 42*: 94–97.

Rokeach, M. 1979. *Understanding Human Values.* New York: The Free Press.

Rosenshine, B., and Furst, N. 1973. The Use of Direct Observation to Study

Teaching. In *Second Handbook of Research on Teaching,* edited by R. Travers, pp. 122–183. Chicago: Rand McNally.

Rosenthal, T.L., and Bandura, A. 1978. Psychological Modeling: Theory and Practice. In *Handbook of Psychotherapy and Behavior Change: An Empirical Analysis,* edited by S.L. Garfield and A.E. Bergin. New York: Wiley.

Rotem, A., and Glasman, M.S. 1979. On the Effectiveness of Student Evaluative Feedback to University Instructors. *Review of Educational Research, 49*: 497–511.

Rous, S.N., Bamford, J.C., Gromisch, D., Rubin, S., and Sall, S. 1972. The Improvement of Faculty Teaching through Evaluation: A Follow-up Report. *Journal of Surgical Research, 13*: 262–266.

Rowe, M.B. 1974. Wait-Time and Rewards as Instructional Variables. *Journal of Research in Science, 11*: 81–84.

Russell, I.J., Caris, T.N., Harris, G.D., and Hendricson, W.D. 1983. Effects of Three Types of Lecture Notes on Medical Student Achievement. *Journal of Medical Education, 58*: 627–636.

Russell, I.J., Hendricson, W.D., Williams, D., and Herbert, R.J. 1984. Effects of Lecture Density on Medical Student Achievement. *Journal of Medical Education, 59*: 881–889.

Sahakian, W.S. 1984. *Introduction to the Psychology of Learning.* Itasca, IL: F.E. Peacock.

Schneider, W., and Shiffrin, R.M. 1977. Controlled and Automatic Human Information Processing: I. Detection, Search, and Attention. *Psychological Review, 84*: 1–66.

Schwenk, T.L., and Whitman, N.A. 1984. *Residents as Teachers: A Guide to Educational Practice.* Salt Lake City: University of Utah School of Medicine.

Seldin, P. 1980. *Successful Faculty Evaluation Programs.* Crugers, NY: Coventry Press.

Sell, G.R. 1986. Perspectives on Peer Review of Teaching in Higher Education. Paper presented at the American Educational Research Association, San Francisco, CA.

Sheehan, J.F., Husted, S.D.R., Candee, D., Cook, C.D., and Bergen, M. 1980. Moral Judgement as a Predictor of Clinical Performance. *Evaluation and the Health Professions, 3*: 393–404.

Sheets, K.J., and Henry, R.C. 1984. Assessing the Impact of Faculty Development Programs in Medical Education. *Journal of Medical Education, 59*(9): 746–748.

Shutz, W. 1966. *The Interpersonal Underworld.* Palo Alto: Science and Behaviors Books.

Sinclair, D.C. 1953. Basic Science—Some Observations in the United States. *Lancet, 1*: 463–467.

Skeff, K.M. 1981. Evaluation of a Method for Improving the Teaching Skills of the Attending Physician. Doctoral dissertation, Stanford University School of Education.

Skeff, K.M. 1983. Evaluation of a Method for Improving the Teaching Performance of the Attending Physician. *American Journal of Medicine, 75*: 465–470.

Skeff, K.M., Campbell, M., and Stratos, B. 1985. Process and Product in Clinical Teaching: A Correlational Study. *Proceedings of the Twenty-Fourth Annual Conference on Research in Medical Education,* pp. 25–29. Washington, DC: Association of American Medical Colleges.

Skeff, K.M., Campbell, M., Stratos, G., Jones, H., and Cooke, M. 1984. Attending Physicians' Assessment of the Seminar Method for Improving Clinical Teaching. *Journal of Medical Education, 59*: 944–950.

Skeff, K.M., and Stratos, G.A. 1985. Two methods for Improving Clinical Teaching: the Intensive Feedback Method and the Seminar Method. *Professions Education Researcher Notes,* 7(2): 6–7.

Skeff, K.M., Stratos, G., Campbell, M., Cooke, M., and Jones, H. 1986. The Evaluation of the Seminar Method to Improve Clinical Teaching. *Journal of General Internal Medicine, 1,* 315–322.

Skinner, B.F. 1938. *The Behavior of Organisms: An Experimental Analysis.* Englewood Cliffs, NJ: Prentice-Hall.

Skinner, B.F. 1957. *Verbal Behavior.* New York: Appleton.

Slamecka, N.J. and Graf, P. 1978. The Generation Effect: Delineation of a Phenomenon. *Journal of Experimental Psychology: Human Learning and Memory, 4*: 592–604.

Sprinthall, N.A., and Thies-Sprinthall, L. 1983. The Teacher as an Adult Learner: A Cognitive-Developmental View. In *Staff Development,* edited by G.A. Griffin. Chicago: The National Society for the Study of Education.

Steiner, W. R. 1935. Reminiscences of Sir William Osler as my Teacher and of my Hospital Experiences Under Him at Johns Hopkins. *Transactions of the American Clinical and Climatological Association, 51*: 51–62.

Stenchever, M.A., Irby, D.M., and O'Toole, B. 1979. A National Survey of Undergraduate Teaching in Obstetrics and Gynecology. *Journal of Medical Education, 54*: 467–470.

Stillman, P.L., Gillers, M.A., Heins, M., Nicholson, G., and Sabers, D.L. 1983. Effect of Immediate Student Evaluations on a Multi-Instructor Course. *Journal of Medical Education, 58*: 173–178.

Stritter, F.T. 1983. Faculty Evaluation and Development. In *Handbook of Health Professions Education,* edited by C.H. McGuire, R.P. Foley, A. Gorr, and R.W. Richards, pp. 294–318. San Francisco: Jossey-Bass.

Stritter, F.T., and Flair, M.D. 1980. *Effective Clinical Teaching.* (PB81-162794) Bethesda, MD: National Medical Audiovisual Center.

Stritter, F.T., Hain, J.D., and Grimes, D.A. 1975. Clinical Teaching Reexamined. *Journal of Medical Education, 50*: 876–882.

Stuart, J., and Rutherford, R.J.D. 1978. Medical Student Concentration During Lectures. *Lancet, 2*: 514–516.

Sweeney, J.M. and Grasha, A.F. 1978. Improving Teaching through Faculty Development Triads. *Improving College and University Teaching Yearbook.* Corvallis, OR: Oregon State University Press.

Thomas, E.J. 1972. The Variation of Memory with Time for Information Appearing During a Lecture. *Studies in Adult Education, 1*: 57–62.

Tremonti, L.B., and Biddle, W.B. 1982. Teaching Behaviors of Residents and Faculty Members. *Journal of Medical Education, 57*: 854–59.

Trower, P., Bryant, B., and Argyle, M. 1978. *Social Skills and Mental Health*. London: Methuen.

Waldrop, M.M. 1984. The Necessity of Knowledge. *Science, 223*: 1279–1282.

Watson, J.B. 1924. *Behaviorism*. New York: W.W. Norton.

Weiner, B. 1980. *Human Motivation*. New York: Holt, Rinehart, & Winston.

Weinholtz, D. 1981. A Study of Instructional Leadership during Medical Attending Rounds. Doctoral dissertation. Chapel Hill: University of North Carolina.

Weinholtz, D. 1983. Directing Medical Student Clinical Case Presentations. *Medical Education, 17*: 364–368.

Weinholtz, D., Albanese, M.A., Zeitler, R. Everett, G., and Shymansky, J. 1986a. Effective Attending Physician Teaching: The Correlation of Observed Instructional Activities and Learner Ratings of Teaching Effectiveness. *Proceedings of the Twenty-fifth Annual Conference On Research In Medical Education, 25*: 273–278.

Weinholtz, D., Everett, G., Albanese, M.A., and Shymansky, J. 1986b. The Attending Round Observation System: A Procedure for Describing Teaching During Attending Rounds. *Evaluation and the Health Professions, 9*: 75–89.

Weinholtz, D., Everett, G., and Shymansky, J. 1985a. Improving Clinical Teaching Through Extensive Observation and Intenstive Feedback. *Professions Education Researcher Notes, 7*(2): 4–6.

Weinholtz, D., Freeman, R.M., and Waickman, L.A. 1986c. Factors Influencing Teaching During Attending Rounds. *Professions Education Researcher Notes, 7*(4): 3–4.

Weinholtz, D., and Friedman, C.P. 1985b. Conducting Qualitative Studies Using Theory and Previous Research: A Study Reexamined. *Evaluation and the Health Professions, 8*: 149–176.

Weinholtz, D., Friedman, C.P., and Watson, E.R. 1985c. A Developmental Model for Teaching in Experiential Learning Settings. *Professions Education Researcher Notes, 6*(4): 3–6.

Weinstein, M.C. and Fineberg, H.V. 1980. *Clinical Decision Analysis*. Philadelphia: Saunders.

Wergin, J.F., Mason, E.J., and Munson, P.J. 1976. The Practice of Faculty Development: An Experience-Derived Model. *Journal of Higher Education, 47*: 289–308.

White, B.Y. 1983. Sources of Difficulty in Understanding Newtonian Dynamics. *Cognitive Science, 7*: 41–65.

Whitman, N.A. 1983. *There is No Gene for Good Teaching: A Handbook on Lecturing for Medical Teachers*. Salt Lake City: University of Utah School of Medicine.

Whitman, N. and Ferrey, A. 1986. Effective Medical Teaching as Characterized by Medical School Teaching Award Winners. Paper delivered at the annual meeting of the American Educational Research Association, San Franciso.

Wilkerson, L. 1985. Learning in a Clinical Setting. *To Improve the Academy, 3:* 120–133. (Accompanying videotape, *Clinical Learning,* available through Health Sciences Consortium)

Wilkerson, L., Lesky, L.G., and Medio, F.J. 1986. The Resident as Teacher on Work Rounds. *Journal of Medical Education, 61*: 823–829.

Wittrock, M.C., 1986. Students' Thought Processes. In *Handbook of Research on Teaching,* edited by M.C. Wittrock. New York: Macmillan.

Yates, F.A. 1966. *The Art of Memory*. London: Routledge and Kegan Paul.

Yelon, S.L., 1973. *Teaching Complex Psychomotor Skills.* East Lansing, MI: Office of Medical Education, Research and Development, Michigan State University.

Appendixes

APPENDIX I
SELF-ASSESSMENT INVENTORY FOR CLINICAL AND CLASSROOM TEACHING IN MEDICINE

OFFICE OF RESEARCH IN MEDICAL EDUCATION
School of Medical Education
University of Washington, Seattle, Washington

DIRECTIONS for Part I: Teacher Behaviors
In this inventory there are statements which reflect some of the ways clinical instructors can be described. For EACH statement, circle the number on the scale which indicates how DESCRIPTIVE the behavior is of your teaching. The scale ranges from 1 for not at all descriptive to 7 for very descriptive. Check (✓) if the behavior is not applicable to the type of teaching you do.

In rating your teaching, respond to each item carefully and thoughtfully. Avoid letting your response to some items influence your responses to others.

Teacher Behaviors	Not at all Descriptive						Very Descriptive	Not Applicable
A. Organization/Clarity								
1. Summarizes major points	1	2	3	4	5	6	7	( )
2. Explains clearly	1	2	3	4	5	6	7	( )
3. Communicates what is expected to be learned	1	2	3	4	5	6	7	( )
4. Presents material in an organized manner	1	2	3	4	5	6	7	( )
5. Emphasizes what is important	1	2	3	4	5	6	7	( )
B. Enthusiasm/Stimulation								
6. Stimulates students'/residents' interest in the subject	1	2	3	4	5	6	7	( )
7. Is enthusiastic about the subject	1	2	3	4	5	6	7	( )
8. Seems to enjoy teaching	1	2	3	4	5	6	7	( )
9. Is a dynamic and energetic person	1	2	3	4	5	6	7	( )
10. Has an interesting style of presentation	1	2	3	4	5	6	7	( )

C. Instructor Knowledge

11. Reveals broad reading in his/her medical specialty . . . . . 1 2 3 4 5 6 7 ( )
12. Directs students/residents to useful literature in the field . . . . . 1 2 3 4 5 6 7 ( )
13. Discusses current developments in his/her specialty . . . . . 1 2 3 4 5 6 7 ( )
14. Demonstrates a breadth of knowledge in medicine generally . . . . . 1 2 3 4 5 6 7 ( )
15. Discusses points of view other than his/her own . . . . . 1 2 3 4 5 6 7 ( )

D. Rapport

16. Provides professional support and encouragement to students/residents . . . . . 1 2 3 4 5 6 7 ( )
17. Establishes rapport with others . . . . . 1 2 3 4 5 6 7 ( )
18. Encourages a climate of mutual respect . . . . . 1 2 3 4 5 6 7 ( )
19. Listens attentively . . . . . 1 2 3 4 5 6 7 ( )
20. Shows a personal interest in students/residents . . . . . 1 2 3 4 5 6 7 ( )
21. Corrects students'/residents' mistakes without belittling them . . . . . 1 2 3 4 5 6 7 ( )
22. Demonstrates sensitivity to the needs of others . . . . . 1 2 3 4 5 6 7 ( )
23. Willingly remains accessible to students/residents . . . . . 1 2 3 4 5 6 7 ( )

E. Instructional Skill

24. Encourages active participation in discussion . . . . . 1 2 3 4 5 6 7 ( )
25. Utilizes audiovisual resources effectively . . . . . 1 2 3 4 5 6 7 ( )
26. Gives students/residents positive reinforcement for good contributions, observations, or performance . . . . . 1 2 3 4 5 6 7 ( )
27. Gears instruction to students'/residents' level of readiness . . . . . 1 2 3 4 5 6 7 ( )
28. Quickly grasps what students/residents are asking or telling . . . . . 1 2 3 4 5 6 7 ( )
29. Answers carefully and precisely questions raised by students/residents . . . . . 1 2 3 4 5 6 7 ( )
30. Questions students/residents to elicit underlying reasoning . . . . . 1 2 3 4 5 6 7 ( )
31. Helps students/residents organize their thoughts about patient problems . . . . . 1 2 3 4 5 6 7 ( )
32. Demonstrates clinical procedures and techniques being taught . . . . . 1 2 3 4 5 6 7 ( )

APPENDIX I (Cont'd)

Teacher Behaviors	Not at all Descriptive						Very Descriptive	Not Applicable
F. Clinical Supervision								
33. Communicates role expectations to students/residents	1	2	3	4	5	6	7	( )
34. Guides students'/residents' development of clinical skills	1	2	3	4	5	6	7	( )
35. Provides specific practice opportunities	1	2	3	4	5	6	7	( )
36. Prepares students/residents for difficult clinical situations	1	2	3	4	5	6	7	( )
37. Offers special help when difficulties arise	1	2	3	4	5	6	7	( )
38. Observes students'/residents' performance frequently	1	2	3	4	5	6	7	( )
39. Identifies students'/residents' strengths and limitations objectively	1	2	3	4	5	6	7	( )
40. Provides frequent feedback on students'/residents' performance	1	2	3	4	5	6	7	( )
41. Makes specific suggestions for improvement	1	2	3	4	5	6	7	( )
42. Seems well prepared for teaching contacts with students/residents	1	2	3	4	5	6	7	( )
43. Questions students/residents in a non-threatening manner	1	2	3	4	5	6	7	( )
G. Clinical Competence								
44. Demonstrates clinical skill and judgment	1	2	3	4	5	6	7	( )
45. Demonstrates skill at data gathering	1	2	3	4	5	6	7	( )
46. Objectively defines patient problems	1	2	3	4	5	6	7	( )
47. Synthesizes patient problems rapidly	1	2	3	4	5	6	7	( )
48. Interprets laboratory data skillfully	1	2	3	4	5	6	7	( )

H. Professional Characteristics

49. Takes responsibility for own actions and procedures	1	2	3	4	5	6	7	( )
50. Recognizes own limitations	1	2	3	4	5	6	7	( )
51. Seems to have self-confidence	1	2	3	4	5	6	7	( )
52. Is self-critical	1	2	3	4	5	6	7	( )
53. Is open-minded and nonjudgmental	1	2	3	4	5	6	7	( )
54. Does not appear to be arrogant	1	2	3	4	5	6	7	( )

Part II: Summary and Action Plan

On the basis of the preceding ratings, circle the numbers on the scales which indicate how descriptive the dimensions of clinical teaching are of your teaching. Check (✓) if the dimension is not applicable to the type of teaching you do.

Dimensions	Not at all Descriptive						Very Descriptive	Not Applicable
A. Organization/Clarity	1	2	3	4	5	6	7	( )
B. Enthusiasm/Stimulation	1	2	3	4	5	6	7	( )
C. Instructor Knowledge	1	2	3	4	5	6	7	( )
D. Rapport	1	2	3	4	5	6	7	( )
E. Instructional Skill	1	2	3	4	5	6	7	( )
F. Clinical Supervision	1	2	3	4	5	6	7	( )
G. Clinical Competence	1	2	3	4	5	6	7	( )
H. Professional Characteristics	1	2	3	4	5	6	7	( )

1. List your strengths in teaching.

2. Describe how you can more effectively capitalize on these strengths.

3. List general areas and specific behaviors of your teaching which need improvement.

   Think about specific situations where the need for improvement was apparent.

5. Outline a plan for improving your teaching:

   A. Teaching behavior: ______________________

      1. New approach:

      2. Assessment procedure:

      3. Summary of results:

B. Teaching behavior: ____________________

1. New approach:

2. Assessment procedure:

3. Summary of results:

APPENDIX II
PEER OBSERVATION FORM FOR CLINICAL TEACHING

Observed ________________ Date ________ Length of Observation ________________

Observer ________________ Setting ________________________

Directions: Components of clinical teaching are listed below to provide a framework for viewing a colleague's instruction. Write specific observations in relation to factors which are appropriate. Use the bottom of the form to summarize strengths and recommendations for improvement.

1. **KNOWLEDGEABLE AND ANALYTICAL** (breadth, analysis and synthesis of ideas)	
2. **ORGANIZATION AND CLARITY OF THOUGHT** (stresses important concepts)	
3. **ENTHUSIASM AND STIMULATION OF INTEREST** (enjoys teaching and profession, dynamic and energetic)	
4. **ESTABLISHES RAPPORT** (shows respect and personal interest in students, listens, supportive)	
5. **COOPERATES WITH OTHER HEALTH CARE PROVIDERS** (communicates and interacts skillfully)	

6. **ACTIVELY INVOLVES LEARNERS** (challenges thought, questions, answers precisely)	
7. **PROVIDES DIRECTION AND FEEDBACK** (guides skill development, observes performance, provides feedback)	
8. **DEMONSTRATES CLINICAL SKILLS AND PROCEDURES** (utilizes skill, judgment and technique)	
9. **PROFESSIONAL CHARACTERISTICS** (self confidence, openness, respect, lack of arrogance, responsibility)	

STRENGTHS:	RECOMMENDATIONS:

APPENDIX III
PEER OBSERVATION FORM FOR CLASSROOM TEACHING

Observed ______________________ Date ______________ Length of Observation ______________

Observer ______________________ Setting ______________________

Directions: Write specific observations in relation to each appropriate factor. Use the bottom of the form to summarize strengths and recommendations for improvement.

CLARITY AND ORGANIZATION

1. Begins by stating importance of topic, objectives, and by previewing main points
2. Presents 2 to 5 main points clearly with supporting examples.
3. Uses instructional resources (eg. slides).
4. Summarizes to achieve closure.

PRESENTATION STYLE

5. Exhibits enthusiasm and stimulates interest in topic.
6. Uses well modulated, clearly articulated speaking voice.
7. Presents without disturbing mannerisms.
8. Paces for note-taking.

GROUP INTERACTION

9. Encourages active participation.
10. Uses questions to challenge thought and stimulate discussion.
11. Responds to questions in clear and non-threatening way.

CONTENT

12. Organizes content logically.
13. Uses up-to-date materials and references.
14. Presents content at appropriate level of complexity and quantity.

HANDOUTS AND EXAMS

15. Prepares appropriate supplementary resources.
16. Examines and grades fairly.

STRENGTHS:	RECOMMENDATIONS:

APPENDIX IV

CLINICAL TEACHING ASSESSMENT FORM UNIVERSITY OF WASHINGTON SCHOOL OF MEDICINE

DEPARTMENT: ______________________ LOCATION: ______________________
YOUR LEVEL: ☐ Resident or ☐ Student DATE: ______________________
DIRECTIONS: Write the name of each faculty member and resident you learned from on this rotation.

Using the teacher behaviors on the right-hand side of the form, rate each faculty member and resident with this scale: 6=Excellent, 5=Very Good, 4=Good, 3=Fair, 2=Poor, 1=Very Poor, and N=Not Applicable.

Avoid letting your responses to some items influence your responses to others.

Add specific behavioral comments regarding strengths and recommendations for improvement in the comments section.

FACULTY, RESIDENTS, ATTENDINGS	Clear and Organized	Enthusiastic/ Stimulating	Establishes Rapport	Actively Involves Students	Knowledgeable/ Analytical	Demonstrates Clinical Skills and Procedures	Provides Direction and Feedback	Accessible	Overall Teaching Effectiveness

NAME: ______________________
COMMENTS:

NAME: ______
COMMENTS:

NAME: ______
COMMENTS:

NAME: ______
COMMENTS:

NAME: ____________
COMMENTS:

NAME: ____________
COMMENTS:

Index